The Transformation of Children's Services

Can we imagine different ways of working together to secure better outcomes for children and families? What are the complex issues that underlie the apparently simple call for 'joined-up' services?

Children's services in many countries around the world are being transformed as part of the call for 'joined-up working for joined-up solutions'. Social, health and educational policy discourses are driven by the idea that 'effective' inter/professional, interagency collaboration is crucial in determining whether service delivery to children and families will succeed or fail. However, the rapid turn from previous inter/professional practices of liaison, consultancy, co-operation and collaboration to more radical and whole-scale service integration and sector transformation has not been accompanied either by a well-considered research agenda of hard questions nor close scrutiny of its effects and consequences.

The book asks a series of searching and challenging questions:

- What are the complex issues involved in children's sector transformation for all those involved – young people, practitioners, leaders and managers, and policy makers?
- How can the 'silos' in which professionals have traditionally been prepared for practice be broken down?
- What are the orthodoxies that surround 'joined-up' working and in what ways should they be challenged?

Written by authors from across the wide range of professional, policy and disciplinary groups involved in this new cross-cutting area of policy and practice, this book provides a critical analysis of the complexities of children's services transformations. The research in this collection addresses the range of discursive, policy and organizational developments associated with the transformation of children's services, providing an important and timely analysis of their complexities, and is essential reading for all those working in the complex spaces of children's services.

Joan Forbes is Senior Lecturer and Director of the Centre for Children's Services Research and Policy Study in the School of Education, University of Aberdeen.

Cate Watson is Senior Lecturer in Professional Learning in the School of Education, University of Stirling.

The Transformation of Children's Services

Examining and debating
the complexities of
inter/professional working

Edited by Joan Forbes
and Cate Watson

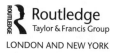 Routledge
Taylor & Francis Group

LONDON AND NEW YORK

First published 2012
by Routledge
2 Park Square, Milton Park, Abingdon, Oxon OX14 4RN

Simultaneously published in the USA and Canada
by Routledge
711 Third Avenue, New York, NY 10017

Routledge is an imprint of the Taylor & Francis Group, an informa business

British Library Cataloguing in Publication Data
A catalogue record for this book is available from the British Library

Library of Congress Cataloging-in-Publication Data
The transformation of children's services: examining and debating the
complexities of inter/professional working/edited by Joan Forbes, Cate Watson.
    p. cm.
    Includes bibliographical references and index.
    1. Children—Services for—Great Britain. 2. Interagency co-ordination—
Great Britain. 3. Children—Services for—United States. 4. Interagency
co-ordination—United States. I. Forbes, Joan. II. Watson, Cate. III. Title.
HV751.A6T73 2011
362.70941—dc22   2011015115

ISBN: 978–0–415–61847–2 (hbk)
ISBN: 978–0–415–61849–6 (pbk)
ISBN: 978–0–203–81841–1 (ebk)

Typeset in Galliard by Keystroke, Station Road, Codsall, Wolverhampton

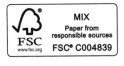

MIX
Paper from
responsible sources
FSC
www.fsc.org   FSC® C004839

Printed and bound in Great Britain by
TJ International Ltd, Padstow, Cornwall

Contents

Contributors

Julie Allan is Professor of Education at the University of Stirling, Scotland, and Visiting Professor at the University of Umeå, Sweden. Her research interests encompass inclusion, children's rights, the arts (especially disability arts) and social capital and she has published widely in these areas. Her most recent books are *Rethinking Inclusive Education: The Philosophers of Difference in Practice* (published by Springer, 2008), *Doing Inclusive Education Research* (with Roger Slee and published by Sense, 2008) and *Social Capital, Professionalism and Diversity* (edited with Jenny Ozga and Geri Smyth and published by Sense, 2009).

John Clarke is a former member of the Centre for Educational Research and Evaluation Services (CERES), Faculty of Education, Leisure and Community, Liverpool John Moores University.

Andrew Cooper is Professor of Social Work at the Tavistock Clinic and the University of East London. He has written and researched widely in the fields of welfare and organizational cultures and on the evolution of the British welfare state including (with Julian Lousada) *Borderline Welfare: Feeling and Fear of Feeling in Modern Welfare*, Karnac Books, 2005.

Michael Cowie is an Honorary Fellow of the College of Humanities and Social Science at the University of Edinburgh. A former head teacher and local authority officer, Michael was previously co-director of the Master's programme in educational leadership and management at the University of Edinburgh. His development work, research interests and publications centre on head teacher preparation and development and school governance.

Megan Crawford is a Reader in Education at Oxford Brookes University where she works with postgraduate students and researches leadership, professional development and innovative assessment.

Gary Crow is Professor of Educational Leadership and Policy Studies at Indiana University, USA. His research interests include work socialization of school site leaders, school leadership and school reform. Gary is currently conducting research on successful school principals and the professional identity of school leaders in reform contexts.

Andrew Eccles is Lecturer in the School of Applied Social Sciences at the University of Strathclyde. His interests lie in the policy contexts of inter/professional working, having conducted research and evaluations for local authorities and health boards in this area, and in ethical issues arising from the use of assistive technologies in community care.

Joan Forbes is Senior Lecturer and Director of the Centre for Children's Services Research and Policy Study, University of Aberdeen. Her research interests are in practitioner knowledges and identities and social and other capitals in schools' and children's services. She edits the *Research Papers* series published by the University of Aberdeen and, with Cate Watson, edited *Service Integration in Schools: Research and Policy Discourses, Practices and Future Prospects* (Sense, 2009).

Walter Humes is a Visiting Professor of Education at the University of Stirling. He has previously held professorships at the universities of Strathclyde, Aberdeen and West of Scotland. His publications include work on teacher education, educational leadership and management, history of education and policy studies. Along with Professor Tom Bryce of Strathclyde University he is co-editor of *Scottish Education*, the 3rd edition of which was published by Edinburgh University Press in 2008.

Ian B. Kerr is a Consultant Psychiatrist and Psychotherapist and member of the Royal College of Psychiatrists, of the British Association of Psychotherapists (Jungian Analytic) and of the Association for Cognitive Analytic Therapy. His clinical and research interests include working with severe and complex 'personality' type disorders and, increasingly, in the social dimensions of mental health and well-being.

Julie McAdam is a Teacher Educator at the School of Education, University of Glasgow. Her research interests include teacher identity and threshold concepts in education. She contributed to *Threshold Concepts in the Disciplines* (Sense, 2009). She is currently involved in an international project on the use of picture books with immigrant children.

James McGonigal is Emeritus Professor of English in Education in the University of Glasgow. He has published national curriculum development materials in language education and support for learning, and has published academic research on classroom interaction, teacher development, literature in learning, and identity and language issues among asylum-seeking children in Scottish schools.

Mark Smith is Lecturer in Social Work in the School of Social and Political Science at the University of Edinburgh. Previously, he was a practitioner and manager in residential child care settings for almost 20 years.

Ian Stronach is Professor of Educational Research and co-director of the Centre for Research and Evaluation Services (CERES) at Liverpool John Moores University, having previously been Research Professor at Manchester Metropolitan University. He is a former editor of the *British Educational Research Journal*. His most recent book is *Globalizing Education, Educating the Local: How Method Made us Mad* (Routledge, 2010).

Cate Watson is Senior Lecturer in the School of Education, University of Stirling, UK. Her main research interests are in professional/institutional identities, leadership and innovative research methodologies. She is the author of *Reflexive Research and the (Re)turn to the Baroque. (Or How I Learned to Stop Worrying and Love the University)*, published by Sense, 2008. With Joan Forbes she edited *Service Integration in Schools: Research and Policy Discourses, Practices and Future Prospects* (Sense, 2009).

Acknowledgements

This book arises out of an ESRC funded seminar series entitled *The effects of professionals' human and cultural capital for interprofessional social capital: exploring professional identities, knowledges and learning for inter-practitioner relationships and interprofessional practice in schools and children's services*, held at the universities of Aberdeen, Glasgow and Strathclyde during 2008–9.

'For whom the bell tolls: education, care and the possibility of professional practice in uncertain times' by Ian Stronach and John Clarke: an earlier version of this chapter appeared in a special issue of the *International Review of Qualitative Research* (2011). The authors of this chapter wish to thank colleagues in the Centre for Educational Research and Evaluation Services (CERES), Liverpool John Moores University, for their helpful comments in our research writing group: Patrick Carmichael, Chandrika Devarokonda (Chester), Alan Hodkinson (now Liverpool Hope University), Marion Jones, Lizzie Smears and Grant Stanley.

Part I

Introduction

Chapter 1

Introducing the complexities of inter/professional working

Joan Forbes and Cate Watson

Introduction

This book is premised on the idea that children's services transformations, currently happening in the UK and many other countries around the globe, are inherently and inescapably characterized by complexity. The title of this book is therefore likely to resonate forcefully with those concerned with such transformations. Clearly, an urgent need exists to uncover and examine these complexities in order to understand better the nature of current transformations. Further, new ways of conceptualizing children's services policy and practice are vital if transformations are to bring benefits to children, young people and their families. This volume explores the view that complexities are inherent in the assumptions underlying both current and proposed future policy and practice in interdisciplinary and transprofessional working across children's services, and, importantly, are produced as an effect of the current professional preparation of practitioners and leaders across the different sectors involved in children's public services. The aim of this volume is therefore to provide a series of alternative perspectives that respect and draw on the diverse knowledges, skills and experiences of those from across the professions involved, in order to examine and encourage debate around the complexities of inter/professional working.

Children's sector transformation, and concomitant remodelling of the sector workforce, has constituted an important and significant recent example of 'travelling policy' across the globe (Lindblad and Popkewitz 2004). Policy imperatives have initiated major service redesign initiatives across children's public services including, for example, recent important work in the UK countries and in the US around full-service schools, extended children's services and children's workforce remodelling. In the United States the No Child Left Behind Act of 2001 (US Congress 2002) initiated and supported a raft of key reforms around service redesign; and in England a programme of reform of children's services was instituted, driven by the Children Act 2004, usually referred to as the *Every Child Matters* agenda (HM Treasury 2003; DfES 2005; DCSF 2008). In Scotland, *Getting it Right for Every Child* (SE 2005) recommends a unified approach to children's services; and in Wales, *A Fair Future for our Children* (WAG 2005) advocates a similar strategy. In Northern Ireland, a strategy for an integrated service agenda for children and young people has been developed around an Extended Schools initiative and implemented in the context of a substantial review of education and public administration (DE 2005; OFMDFM

2006); while Eire has developed a parallel agenda driven by the *Giving Children an Even Break* policy (IE 2001). In these and other polities globally, the redesign of children's services policy and governance has been characterized by the idea that 'effective' inter/professional interagency collaboration is crucial in determining whether services to children and families will succeed or fail.

What holds these different programmes and agendas together is a widely shared and almost unquestioned belief that interagency collaboration is a very good thing and that more of it is needed. Inter/professional practice appears to be a holy grail, thought capable of delivering 'effectiveness' and 'excellence' in even the most challenging of circumstances (Brown 2009; Pugh 2009). Moving beyond better co-ordinated services and greater co-operation has, however, proved problematic. Evaluative reports into children's services redesign have suggested that practitioners find it difficult to translate the concepts of collaboration and partnership into practice (Sammons *et al.* 2002, 2003a, 2003b; Allan, Mannion and Duffield 2004; Whitty and Campbell 2004). Practitioners have been described as allowing little cross-fertilization (Power *et al.* 2003), being 'relatively entrenched in their attitudes' and having 'not deviated or altered their way of doing things that much' (Sammons *et al.* 2003a: 71). That these problems stubbornly persist despite repeated injunctions to collaborate suggests the need for a critical examination of the changing discourses concerning co-practice in the children's sector in policy, and of the effects of any new recommendations for closer or integrated practice.

The debate presented in this book around the new and different kinds of theoretical and conceptual frameworks that are required to adequately take account of the complexities in transformation is therefore timely. Critical examination of the many intertwined components of transformation is urgently needed to consider implications for: inter/transprofessional workforce 'remodelling'; new work relations; and children's services locations. Questioning the preparation of practitioners and, crucially, the role of leadership and management in integrated children's services, is also vital. This collection therefore fulfils a critical need to analyse the impact of the transformation of children's services on professional identities and changing knowledge, practice and power relations; and to present new analytics that can more fully grasp and make sense of the fluid, uncertain and less predictable kinds of professional relationships necessitated by, and emerging as a result of, the integration of children's services.

The book arises out of an ESRC-funded seminar series entitled *The effects of professionals' human and cultural capital for interprofessional social capital: Exploring professional identities, knowledges and learning for inter-practitioner relationships and interprofessional practice in schools and children's services*, held at the universities of Aberdeen, Glasgow and Strathclyde during 2008–9. The seminars aimed to explore a number of important questions arising from new professional relations in moves towards children's services integration in the UK and globally. Important themes addressed in this collection therefore include:

- policy, theory and discourses surrounding inter/professional practice;
- the formation of professional identities and their impact on inter/professional practice;

- the role of early professional training and socialization into professional norms, values and roles;
- the effects of the complex relationships between professionals' identities, knowledge and practice in the development of practitioners' social and other capitals;
- critical questioning of the assumptions that underlie current and future practice in schools and children's services to uncover and question what now needs to change or be done differently if future services to children and young people are to be made better.

The core theme for the book is transformations in children's services, in particular in relation to the role played by schools and the education service in the children's sector nexus. Within this core theme the book falls into three main sections. The first two examine respectively the complexities of inter/professional working and preparation for practice, while the third questions current orthodoxies surrounding notions of collaborative working. A major strength of this collection is the range of contributors – from health, social work and education – and a corresponding wide range of theoretical perspectives which aim to open up and stimulate debate across, and within, disciplines and professions. The book balances theoretical chapters with contributions which draw on empirical work and practice. It draws on specific case studies, recognizing that the global field for children's services transformations makes the cases studied relevant to the wider UK context and beyond. Mindful that examinations and debates concerning current transformations in children's sector services are of global interest and concern, the book includes contributions of significant interest to an international audience from academics and children's public sector practitioners from across the UK countries and the USA.

Following the introduction, Part II is entitled *Policy, theory, discourse: the complexities of collaborative working.* This sets out and examines the policy context/s within which calls for 'joined-up' working are located. Andrew Cooper's chapter identifies a number of critical current challenges for those working in the children's public sector and the implications of these are taken up in subsequent chapters. In Chapter 3, Andrew Eccles argues that our understanding of 'collaboration' must be informed by an understanding of the politics of partnership. In Chapter 4, Joan Forbes stresses the need for close attention to potential points of policy-practice tension, incoherence or disconnect in the current redesign of transprofessional relations. Finally, in Chapter 5, Ian Stronach and John Clarke, questioning the spurious certainties of the economic and financial market epistemologies which have infiltrated education and children's sector social policy, urge a turn to an epistemology of uncertainty more fitting to the difficulties and risks involved in education and children's services work in the current moment.

Andrew Cooper's opening chapter, introducing the contemporary challenges of working together, acts as an initial thoughtful provocation for the examinations and debates in the chapters that follow. He carefully sets out the context within which calls for joined-up working are situated. In particular, Cooper considers a number of assumptions surrounding 'collaborative working' with the intention of stimulating deeper debate on issues relating to inter/professional working and the character of modern public sector organizations. The chapter deftly considers the problems and possibilities of inter/professional working in human service organizations, and children's services in particular, in terms of an interaction between the task to be carried out, the professionals charged with this, and the complex systems and organizations within which they are asked to carry out their work. Each of these layers, Cooper argues, has its own particular associated tensions that render the task of inter/professional working possible – but difficult. Cooper concludes that the development of new organizational structures in the public sector aimed at producing more fluid and networked forms of working do support the emergence of innovative approaches, but equally these developments present threats to professional identity that must be understood if we are to overcome them, a key theme that is taken up and responded to by contributors throughout the book.

In Chapter 3, Andrew Eccles responds to Cooper's provocation that meta-level analyses which provide understandings of policy and governance are now needed in his examination of political aspects of the growth of partnership working in children's public services across the United Kingdom polities. Over the past ten years a burgeoning literature has developed around the idea of partnerships, their operation and processes of policy delivery, as a central feature of government thinking. There has, however, been less specific discussion about the complexities of the *politics* of partnership working. The political considerations addressed here include the ideological framework in which partnerships have evolved, an examination of the policy-making process itself and – often underestimated – the politics of implementation. An overarching concern is the question of political power and its dynamics: who might hold it and how it might be exercised in the complex realities of partnership working. The analysis presented here, which considers *inter alia* how policy has emerged, tensions between central and local government, and between policy and practice, draws largely on the experience of Scotland, which, in its post-devolution guise, has seen particularly concerted attempts by government to change relationships between education, health and social care through partnership working across these sectors.

Taking up and developing the theme of policy-practice power relations, in Chapter 4 Joan Forbes analyses the redesign of professional relations, or *transprofessional capital*, in the current policy trajectories of children's services. She discusses recent policies in the UK countries and other places predicated on the notion that public services for children and young people need to work better together to be effective at all levels if the aims of social and educational inclusion are to be achieved. With this as a starting point she takes as a case study some of the inconsistencies in Scottish education and allied health professions policy which produce policy-practice disjunctures for those involved. Forbes draws on social capital theory and presents a mapping of social capital interstices as a conceptual and analytical framework to discern and explore these potential disjunctures in practice relations between education and allied health professions practitioner groups, theorizing this as an effect of their particular stocks of human capital formed in specific mono-subject disciplinary knowledge practices. Using published data concerning education and the allied health professions as exemplification, the chapter analyses the ways in which the social capital resources held and used by these two groups of children's sector practitioners, their *transprofessional* and *transdisciplinary capital,* currently work effectively or break down in policy-practice incoherence and inherent disconnects in transprofessional social capital-in-practice. Forbes concludes that children's sector integration may not solve previous problems and may indeed create new problems to do with size and complexity that are too hard to manage. But in either case, she maintains that new conceptualizations and analytics are urgently needed to examine the materiality of the forms of practitioner relations as these are done, blocked or fudged in cross-boundary trans-sectoral integration-in-practice.

Part II ends with Ian Stronach and John Clarke's theoretical insights into the nature and effects of current education discourses, including those surrounding the transformation of children's services. The thesis informing this chapter is that the future of children's services needs to embrace a new epistemology of uncertainty. Stronach and Clarke argue that prior to the 2008 Crash the scientificist certainty of 'financial engineering' migrated into the discourses and methodologies of education and health. Across the (children's) public sector, economistic and statistical metaphors were appropriated – markets, measurement of inputs/outputs, audit, accountability, league tables and the 'knowledge economy'. Stronach and Clarke argue that econo-mizing assumptions and a world view commodifying the social and the educational became accepted in/through the available economic epistemology, discourses and metaphors, e.g., those of social, cultural and other 'capitals', but that as global and financial markets crashed in 2008, the certainties – albeit always fantasies – of financial/economic epistemologies and the order, progress and predictability of the 'knowledge economy' vanished with them. The chapter ends with the warning that scientific capitalism and its underlying philosophy, although illusory and discredited in the Crash, will mutate and re-invade the public sector – and perhaps has already done so. In response, Stronach and Clarke conclude with an appeal to the merit of an epistemology of uncertainty more appropriate to the risks involved in the unruliness and disruption which attend current efforts to theorize and conceptualize children's services discourses and practices.

The next part of the book, *Preparing practitioners and leaders for inter/professional practice: identities, connections, knowledges,* focuses on inter/professional practice and the education, training and preparation of professionals for this. In Chapter 6, James McGonigal and Julie McAdam examine 'threshold concepts' as conceptual gateways or portals which must be understood by early career professionals in the development of inter/professional working. In Chapter 7, Michael Cowie and Megan Crawford discuss issues arising from a case study of the development of primary head teachers working within the context of schools/children's services. In Chapter 8, Gary Crow highlights the complexity of inter/professional working and what is required to train leaders in education to undertake this. Finally in this part, Chapter 9, by Ian Kerr considers the limitations inherent in current, competing models adopted by different professionals working within mental health care provision and presents a case study of an integrated approach aimed at providing a common understanding among such professionals.

In Chapter 6, James McGonigal and Julie McAdam closely examine the question of how practitioners might be better equipped for inter/professional practice. They start from the premise that if effective inter/professional working is to develop between those who work with children and young people in various educational and care contexts, then some sort of shared 'theory' is needed. Theory here is taken to mean a rationale that is assented to by the different professionals involved in such working together, and a felt awareness of the attitudes, values and constraints that operate within their different contexts. McGonigal and McAdam argue that social capital theory offers one perspective, providing a framework for thinking about the relational dimensions of inter/professional practice, but because social capital as theory is more effectively deployed at the macro-level of policy or the meso-level of reflection, rather than at the micro-level of practice, additional theory is needed to maximize its potential in exploring the complex realities of professional decision-making. To address these concerns, McGonigal and McAdam introduce a potentially fruitful theory, fresh in its application to inter/professional relations, but one that is currently used to think about conceptual difficulties and, increasingly, professional learning across a range of academic disciplines. The notion of *troublesome knowledge* and of *threshold concepts* as 'conceptual gateways' enabling perceptual shifts in the development of professionals' knowledges can perhaps offer a shared language in which the next generation of teachers and social workers can begin to understand each others' aims and intentions.

Taking up and addressing the theme of the preparation of professionals, the contribution by Michael Cowie and Megan Crawford goes deeper in analysing leadership learning for practice in and through the Scottish Qualification for Headship (SQH) programme. The chapter emerges from an International Study of the Preparation of Principals (ISPP), conducted in ten countries. It discusses the outcomes of three linked studies on the experience of professional socialization as reported by a small group of primary head teachers. The empirical work on which this analysis draws was designed to explore the utility of formal preparation programmes to novice head teachers. For Cowie and Crawford, and their colleagues in the ISPP study, this has involved understanding how newly appointed heads make sense of headship and how well they perceive they have been prepared for managing and leading schools and children's services. Crucially, Cowie and Crawford investigate how the new heads say they enacted and developed their understanding of headship through time. Emerging from the central theme of leadership preparation, the chapter examines a range of issues relating to the complexities of inter/professional socialization, inter/professional identity and the purposes of head teacher preparation in the current context of the transformation of schools and children's services.

Gary Crow's chapter continues this theme and addresses more closely the questions of leadership education and preparation, characterized here as the making of inter/professional leaders for inter/professional practice. He highlights the complexity of inter/professional working and what is required to form and equip leaders in education to undertake this. Specifically, the chapter sets out to examine the concept of professional identities of school leaders. Crow's aim is to encourage a conversation about the importance of professional identity for school leadership practice, in particular the leader's role in inter/professional collaboration. To accomplish this, the chapter first explores the changing nature of work in post-industrial society and the importance of professional identity for one aspect of this work – inter/professional practice. Second, it examines what Crow believes is an unfortunate trend in which professional identity is being ignored in favour of a more technical orientation to the role of school leader. Third, the chapter explores the concept of professional identity – its definitions, importance and development, drawing on an empirical study to identify elements of head teachers' socialization that aims to contribute to an understanding of the development of professional identity among school leaders. Finally, the chapter identifies some implications of the development of professional identity for strengthening inter/professional practice.

Issues of mental health and well-being are central to a consideration of the provision of integrated services for children and young people (see, for example, Shucksmith *et al.* 2005). The concluding chapter in Part III by Ian Kerr draws on the premise that current models of professional work in mental health are informed by a number of 'competing' and sometimes conflicting paradigms. These range from the bio-medical, to the psychological through to the more exclusively socio-economic. Kerr argues, however, that to create an adequate and culturally sensitive conceptualization of mental health and social problems, more genuinely integrative and developmental models are required that address the issue of how, in a dialectical process, specific factors determine and shape the so-called 'psychopathology' of individuals in a given society, and how these societal factors are in turn shaped by individuals. Without adequate and, crucially, *shared* models, Kerr argues, any attempt at individual intervention may render futile attempts to help or heal 'individuals'. It may also, importantly, lead to disagreements, arguments, stress and 'burn out' amongst the practitioners involved – whatever their professional identifications. Seeking to address such challenges, this chapter examines a pilot project offering a basic training to a professionally mixed community mental health team in cognitive-analytic therapy (CAT). This model provides a common language to acknowledge and describe 'socio-psychopathology' and its individual expression. His analysis of the CAT model leads the author to conclude that it may offer a timely intervention agenda to help children's services practitioners to focus more clearly and collectively on the task, increase team cohesion and morale and reduce stress and 'burn out'.

Part IV, *Questioning the orthodoxies of collaboration*, sets out to uncover and challenge unexamined assumptions that inform inter/professional working across the children's services sector. In Chapter 10, Mark Smith examines the way in which current policy in social work has resulted in the 'fragmentation' of the child and suggests that European models of 'social pedagogy' might produce more fruitful ways of working. In Chapter 11, Julie Allan focuses on higher education and considers the tensions between the academy and the professions it prepares. Cate Watson presents a 'fictional case study' in Chapter 12 as a means to illustrate the way in which organizations undermine the efforts of individuals to engage in collaborative working. Finally, in Chapter 13, Walter Humes draws the threads of this section together and asks whether there are limits to collaboration.

Part IV opens with Mark Smith's chapter which takes as its point of departure the assumption that social work, conceived at the height of modernist optimism, has fallen prey to postmodern fragmentation, anxiety and pessimism. This fragmentation can be applied, too, at a conceptual level. The 'whole child' model of social education or 'upbringing' envisaged by Kilbrandon (1964) and evident in European social pedagogy, has been crowded out by the intellectually and morally restricting discourses of rights and protection. Smith argues that aspirations for children are best served within broadly educational approaches to practice rather than those rooted in individual or family deficit or blame, which seem to be embedded within dominant Anglo-American paradigms of social welfare. Reflecting that discursive shifts from welfare towards a dominant neoliberal consumerism have also taken their toll on professional identities, Smith emphasizes that while social workers may still come into the profession determined to make a difference in people's lives they are ground down in a petty proceduralism that dissipates this initial moral purpose. In a careful and detailed analysis, the author demonstrates that the social work profession is currently conflicted by internal tensions where daily practice is dissonant with espoused values. Concluding that we have reached a stage where social work is neither 'social', nor is it working, Smith calls for this disconnection not to be viewed as an insoluble predicament; rather it should serve as a provocation which opens up spaces to reclaim some of social work's broadly educational roots.

Chapter 11, by Julie Allan, examines the role of the university educator in the development of professionals. Starting from a critique of the ways in which the preparation and role of the academic within universities has become increasingly constrained by the 'audit culture', Allan argues that what academics write and for whom is more closely circumscribed than ever before, and the pressure to demonstrate 'impact', whatever that may be, limits their capacity to have any real influence on communities and on their values. Allan argues that the culture of audit in the current university does impact on initial professional education, however, resulting in programmes that are highly prescriptive, technicized and surrounded by 'theory junk sculpture' (Thomas 2008), offering little incentive for beginning professionals to make connections with one another. Further, efforts at promoting inter/professional practice, when they are made, are driven not by civic responsibility but by an 'emotivism' (MacIntyre 1999), which, Allan argues, is urged onto others 'under the guise of a well-argued and *moral* evaluation', and ultimately limited by the highly contextualized boundaries of teaching and of other professions. In response to this, Allan argues a need to recapture the civic, proposing a role for academics as the facilitators of 'everyday epiphanies', creating spaces where colleagues and stakeholders in policy and practice communities can come together to 'dwell upon' routine in order to uncover the quality of what is actually experienced in inter/professional work.

Offering a further provocation to prevailing paradigm orthodoxies, Cate Watson's contribution discusses the ways in which, currently, children's services policy is mobilized around the notion of 'joined-up working', which she describes as a 'pretty story' in which policy is offered as a vision of what might be achieved (and hence what could be avoided) if professionals only set aside their selfish self-interest and worked together for children. The pretty story of joined-up working presents as smooth uncontested consensus imposing closure, while simultaneously offering a utopian vision based on *partnership* and *collaboration*. But how does this play out in practice? Watson's chapter sets out to expose the pretty story to scrutiny at the micro level. More especially, the chapter examines the construction, performance and interplay of organizational, institutional and professional identities when staff of different organizations occupy a shared workplace, if not a shared space of practice. The chapter ostensibly presents a 'case study', drawing on interview data from members of staff of two different organizations, a primary school and an agency offering therapeutic services, offered as a partial account which aims to unsettle and subvert unproblematic constructions of joined-up working. Watson concludes by arguing that impediments to joined-up working imposed by the ideology of rationality that pervades organizations frustrate the development of inter/professional capital, and suggests that a similar adherence to this ideology among researchers may also undermine attempts to reconceptualize practice.

Questioning the prevailing orthodoxies of inter/professional collaboration discourses and practices and examining their limits is the focus of the concluding chapter in this part. Walter Humes analyses and challenges the prevailing discourse of collaboration, exemplified in the emphasis on multi-agency working, communities of practice and interdisciplinary research. Illustrating his analysis with critique of examples from the fields of health, education and social work, Humes argues that while such developments are understandable responses to perceived weaknesses in previous modes of operation and forms of provision, there has been insufficient critical scrutiny of their underlying assumptions. Reflecting critically on the considerable attention which has been directed at issues of structure, communication and professional training, the author contends that the potential risks of a 'collective' approach to service provision have been under-examined. Humes concludes that greater conceptual clarity is needed to unpack and examine the underlying constituent features of such a collective model for the transformation of children's services, including the blurring of lines of responsibility, the formation of a 'protectionist' model of professional identity and the marginalizing of important ethical concerns.

Part V, *Conclusion*, features the final chapter *inter/professional children's services: complexities, transformations and futures*, where we conclude that it is through knowledgeable, skilled and experienced practitioners' careful and detailed examination and debate of the complex issues inherent in the design of good services to children that knowledge may be gained about what it is necessary and desirable to hold on to, discard and/or transform. The transformation of children's services in the current moment constitutes a space that is driven by and incorporates a wide number of competing agendas and aspirations. The chapters in this book show that through knowledgeable examination and debate contributed from across the spectrum of alternative professional perspectives the complex challenges of inter/professional working may be opened up to scrutiny and more clearly grasped, so as better to inform future transformation of inter/professional children's services.

References

Allan, J., Mannion, G. and Duffield, J. (2004) 'Premature evaluation? Measuring the impact of Integrated Community Schools', *Scottish Educational Review* 36: 145–58.

Brown, D. (2009) 'Leadership and capacity in the public sector: integrated children's services and schools', in J. Forbes and C. Watson (eds) *Service integration in schools: research and policy discourses, practices and future prospects*, Rotterdam: Sense.

Department for Children, Schools and Families (DCSF) (2008) *2020 Children and young people's workforce strategy*, Nottingham: DCSF.

Department for Education and Skills (DfES) (2005) *Children's workforce strategy*, London: DfES.

Department of Education (DE) (Northern Ireland) (2005) *Draft supplementary guidance to support the impact of SENDO on the Code of Practice on the identification and assessment of special educational needs*, Bangor: DE.

Department of Education (IE) Social Inclusion Unit (2001) *Giving children an even break by tackling disadvantage in primary schools*, Dublin: Department of Education and Science. Online. Available at: http://www.education.ie/home/home.jsp?pcategory=17216and ecategory=34287andlanguage=EN (accessed 7 August 2010).

HM Treasury (2003) *Every child matters*, London: HMSO.

Kilbrandon, Lord C. J. D. Shaw (1964) *The Kilbrandon Report: children and young persons Scotland*, Edinburgh: HMSO. Reprinted 1995. Online. Available at: http://www. scotland.gov.uk/Resource/Doc/47049/0023863.pdf (accessed 14 March 2011).

Lindblad, S. and Popkewitz, T. S. (eds) (2004) *Educational restructuring: international perspectives on travelling policies*, Greenwich: Information Age Publishing.

MacIntyre, A. (1999) *Dependent rational animals: why human beings need the virtues*, Chicago: Open Court Press.

Office of the First Minister and Deputy First Minister (OFMDFM) (2006) *Our children and young people – our pledge. A ten-year strategy for children and young people in Northern Ireland, 2006–2016*, Belfast: OFMDFM.

Power, S., Halpin, D., Whitty, G. and Gewirtz, S. (2003) *Paving a 'Third Way'?: a policy trajectory analysis of Education Action Zones. Research report to Economic and Social Research Council*, London: ESRC.

Pugh, G. (2009) 'Every Child Matters: the implications for service integration in England', in J. Forbes and C. Watson (eds) *Service integration in schools: research and policy discourses, practices and future prospects*, Rotterdam: Sense.

Sammons, P., Power, S., Elliot, K., Robertson, P., Campbell, C. and Whitty, G. (2002) 'National evaluation of the New Community Schools pilot programme in Scotland: phase 1: interim findings', *Interchange 76*, Edinburgh: Scottish Executive Education Department.

Sammons, P., Power, S., Elliot, K., Robertson, P., Campbell, C. and Whitty, G. (2003a) *New Community Schools in Scotland. Final report. National evaluation of the pilot phase*, London: Institute of Education, University of London.

Sammons, P., Power, S., Elliot, K., Robertson, P., Campbell, C. and Whitty, G. (2003b) 'Key findings from the national evaluation of the New Community Schools pilot programme in Scotland', *Insight 7*, Edinburgh: Scottish Executive Education Department.

Scottish Executive (SE) (2005) *Getting it right for every child: proposals for action*, Edinburgh: Scottish Executive.

Shucksmith, J., Philip, K., Spratt, J. and Watson, C. (2005) *Investigating the link between mental health and behaviour in schools*, Edinburgh: SEED.

Thomas, G. (2008) 'Theory and the construction of pathology', paper presented at the American Educational Research Association Conference, New York, USA, 24–8 March.

US Congress (2002) *An Act to close the achievement gap with accountability, flexibility and choice so that no child is left behind*. Washington: US Congress. Online. Available at: http://www.ed.gov/policy/e/sec/leg/esea02/107-110pdf (accessed 20 March 2009).

Welsh Assembly Government (WAG) (2005) *A fair future for our children*, Cardiff: The Welsh Assembly Government. Online. Available at: http://wales.gov.uk/dsjlg/publications/ childrenyoung/fairfuture/strategy?lang=en (accessed 7 August 2010).

Whitty, G. and Campbell, C. (2004) 'Integrating social justice and schooling: research evidence and policy concerns', in J. Forbes (ed.) *Values and vision: working together in Integrated Community Schools?* Aberdeen: University of Aberdeen.

Part II

Policy, theory, discourse

The complexities of collaborative working

Chapter 2

Complexity, identity, failure

Contemporary challenges to working together

Andrew Cooper

Introduction

In this chapter I want to take the liberty of making certain assumptions in order, hopefully, to provoke deeper debate on issues relating to inter/professional working and the character of modern public sector organizations.

Just before I wrote the first version of this chapter I attended one of the seminars which formed part of the review process Lord Laming had been asked by government at Westminster to conduct in the wake of the 'Baby P' (we now know his name was Peter Connelly) case in the London borough of Haringey and other cases across England that caused immense public and political disquiet. [1] We know that difficulties in inter/professional communication and co-operation are the factors most consistently cited in analyses of public inquiries and Serious Case Reviews in relation to the deaths of children over the years (Reder and Duncan 2004). [2] As Reder and Duncan say in their meta-analysis of these documents, 'The consistency between the findings is striking, with particular clusters around: deficiencies in the assessment process; problems with interprofessional communication; inadequate resources; and poor skills acquisition or application' (ibid.: 96).

During the New Labour government era, 1997–2010, a particular public policy culture became established, organized around strong centralized state control of organizational and individual 'performance'. Public service 'failure' was tackled through regimes of inspection, performance management, reward and punishment. Since coming to power in the UK in May 2010 the Conservative–Liberal Democrat coalition government has set about dismantling this vast state apparatus in England. In child protection services the *Munro Review* (Munro 2011) signals a period of de-bureaucratized 'judgement-based' and relationship-based practice. The current government's wider reforms emphasize 'localism', and an aspiration to mobilize voluntary and community resources in place of, or in support of, directly funded provision, sometimes referred to as the 'Big Society' initiative. But the nature of difficult child protection work may not change that much from the perspective of front-line practice – and to the extent that public expectations of public service 'performance' have been raised in the last decade, evidence of 'failures' in this new world may not be as easily forgiven as the political classes seem to hope it will be.

Five dimensions of inter/professional working

I want to consider the problems and possibilities of inter/professional working in human service organizations, and children's services in particular, in terms of an interaction between:

- the task – the nature of the work we do;
- professionals as people;
- professionals as members of complex systems;
- the organizational forms that support or contain these systems; and
- complexity and modern organizational forms.

The main assumption I want to make relates to 'complex systems' in public sector work and the organizational forms in which they are embedded, and my belief that they have become more, not less, complex in recent years. In part this is because we no longer have a simple public–private–independent sector divide. The public sector 'project' in Britain is now enacted via a set of cross-sectoral processes involving all three of these domains, the overall enterprise supposedly held together by another set of processes and principles called 'governance'. The idea of 'governance' reflects the somewhat curious, hybrid character of the modern public sector beast – neither precisely a part of traditional 'government' in the sense of government functioning as a direct provider; yet not quite *not* a part of government, since somebody or some set of processes has to assume overall responsibility for the co-ordination, efficiency and 'fitness for purpose' of the enterprise. Where public sector organizations are not responsible for delivering services, public money is usually funding whoever is doing the providing. So government has only half vacated the scene.

There is much more that could be said about this new order of welfare, but I am interested in a fifth dimension of interaction – the socio-economic environment in which our organizations are located, and the shaping influence of this environment on our daily practice as this is mediated by our organizations and systems. However, perhaps I have already, in a few sentences, made a case for the difficulty of knowing where our organizations begin and end. Who is paying for and who is providing services, in what shifting configuration? Are services now a form of 'provision' or are they, in line with the dominant model of market choice, merely the provision of a structure of 'opportunity' in which the onus is on the rational, active citizen to access these opportunities in pursuit of their chosen welfare outcomes – a decent education, a viable pension plan, good health. The American political theorist Philip Bobbitt has written of the passing of the nation state, and the emergence of the 'market state', and this revised concept of the state extends to the welfare state:

> Bush and Blair . . . are among the first market state political leaders. They appeal to a new standard – whether their policies improve and expand the opportunities offered to the public – because this standard reflects the basis for a new form of the State.
>
> (Bobbitt 2003: 222)

Postmodern contexts – can we cope?

This 'mixed economy' of welfare, in which it seems to be the case that no one agency, let alone one individual, is in single overall control or holds overall responsibility for the functioning of the total enterprise, is the postmodern context of welfare. I will cite one example of how this state of affairs is represented in recent policy literature – a 2008 Commission for Social Care Inspection (CSCI) report on safeguarding adults:

> Despite . . . subsequent development and implementation of local policies and procedures for safeguarding adults, people told us that it is still not clear who has overall accountability. They said that whilst most of the individual pieces of the multi-agency jigsaw seem to exist in one form or another, it is not clear to people how those pieces fit together to form a coherent picture. Nor is it clear which agency has a complete view of that picture.
>
> (CSCI 2008: 10)

Simply stated, we had enough trouble managing our inter/professional and inter-agency relationships in the 'old world' of the bounded traditional organization, so what do we make of the impact of this 'fifth dimension' of complexity? Of course, one person's safe and well-bounded organizational culture may be another's breeding ground for silo mentalities. Paradoxically, one driver producing the fluid, unstable, flexible, loosely bounded organizational culture of postmodern welfare was discontent with our ability to work effectively across these same boundaries. The answer seems to have been to loosen or dissolve the boundaries, enabling more 'integrated' or 'joined-up' working practices. Or is it?

The question at the heart of what I want to discuss takes the form of a tension: the need for strong professional identities on the one hand, and the dangers of these on the other; the need to have boundaries to work across if professional identities are not to become merged, indistinct, meaningless, and the risk of inadvertently producing a kind of fundamentalist backlash as professional groups seek to defend identities they feel to be threatened by the push towards multi-agency, multi-professional working. At a broader level of analysis, the sociologist Anthony Giddens (1994: 85) described fundamentalism as 'tradition defended in the traditional way', alerting us to the existential anxieties mobilized by perceived threats to 'identity'.

I do not want to be excessively pessimistic about our capacity for effective inter/professional relationships; but I do not want to be naïvely optimistic either. Much contemporary policy discourse errs on the side of the latter, blithely assuming that professional identities can and should be discarded or re-fashioned in pursuit of more 'user-focused' services and practices. Often the unspoken message is that these traditional identities had little substantive value in the first place, other than as a means of protecting a set of vested interests. Professional protectionism and self-replication is certainly a problem, but there also may be a deeper value lying within the over-protected 'space' of professional identity that we attack at our peril.

Professional identity and the policy process

At the 2009 seminar with Lord Laming, one widely shared anxiety concerned how professionals in children's services feel they are now being asked to do jobs quite different from the ones they were trained for: teachers feel they are being asked to become social workers; health visitors feel they are front-line child protection staff not preventative health workers; social workers feel like police; and since the last Laming Report (2009) police feel they have become split off from social services and marginalized on the child protection front line. It's a great idea, 'co-locating' social services in schools, but it's the kind of great idea that probably needs three to five years to be really made to work as staff from all locations adjust and learn.

There is always something impatient, hasty, pushy about policy change processes – and then, when change doesn't happen as magically and rapidly as the politicians and policy makers are willing it to happen, something complex occurs: professional groups are accused of being resistant, inward-looking, dependent, conservative, and of guarding their vested interests. Maybe they are, but maybe also they are manifesting something ordinary, that needs respect – they are manifesting conflict about change, conflict about what they are being asked to give up that is valued by them, and may well have been of value to the people they serve. 'Resistance to organizational change' is one of those phrases that we often deploy in a lazy, thoughtless manner. Psycho-analytic models of organizational dynamics have perhaps colluded with this, but my colleague William Halton at the Tavistock Clinic has written about how we need the capacity to distinguish between resistance to change on the one hand and the desire to fight to preserve something valuable that is under attack on the other (Halton 2004). Strong professional identities have evolved not only for defensive and narcissistic reasons; they have evolved in the context of practitioners, researchers, professional teachers and trainers, and theorists all collaborating intensively over long periods of time in pursuit of better ways of doing the job, whatever that may be – teaching, doctoring, health visiting and so on.

The context of failure

The imperative towards developing better inter/professional and inter-organizational working seems to be in danger of forgetting this. Why? Well, one important reason is what I will call the 'context of failure'. I have alluded to what is well known to all of us – that in England, children's service and child protection policy in particular has been driven by a perverse process in which about once every five years a significant 'failure' is surfaced in the public domain – never mind that similar 'failures' are happening all the time if anyone cared to concern themselves between times – and this 'failure' becomes the occasion of massive public, political and professional hand-wringing; hasty, panicky, anxiety-driven change is usually the result. The drive to improve and develop inter/professional working is caught up in this process. One can hardly be against 'joined-up working' like it's hard to be in favour of sin; but it can be galling to feel, first, that one may have already been practising it very effectively on the quiet for many years, and, second, (paradoxically) that we are being herded towards it rather like naughty children who have misbehaved by not talking enough to one another in class – something that 'teacher' has just noticed though it has been going on for years.

If this sounds contradictory, then maybe it is. We can be both very good at working together, and terrible at doing so. What is for certain, given the repetitive findings of 30 years of public inquiries into the worst consequences of us not talking and working together properly, is that despite best efforts we seem not to be very good at improving on the situation. Why might this be? I want to discuss two kinds of answer – these are not the whole of the story, just some less often noticed and discussed aspects of the picture.

The task

First of all, the nature of the task; one of the consequences of policy change being driven so much by episodes of professional 'failure' is that attention becomes almost exclusively directed towards those who are held to have failed, and the systems within which they function. Attention is directed away from the nature of the task in relation to which we are deemed to have failed – the task of protecting children or working to improve the conditions of life of children with complex needs. You cannot protect children at risk without engaging with their families. And the fact is that a small, but very significant, minority of these families are just exceptionally difficult to engage with. A whole series of (in principle) avoidable professional mistakes and oversights underlay the deaths of both Victoria Climbié and Peter Connelly but Lord Laming in his first Inquiry Report did have this to say:

> Staff doing this work need a combination of professional skills and personal qualities, not least of which are persistence and courage. Adults who deliberately exploit the vulnerability of children can behave in devious and menacing ways. They will often go to great lengths to hide their activities from those concerned for the well being of a child.
>
> (DHHO 2003: 3)

At a seminar I attended around the time of the publication of that report I heard a senior manager in a social work agency express this rather more graphically. 'Look,' she said, 'many of the adults we have to deal with in child abuse cases are complete bastards'.

Government commissioned research into serious case reviews between 2003 and 2005 (Brandon *et al.* 2008) found that only 12 per cent of the children killed or injured were on the Child Protection Register. In other words, nearly 90 per cent of the most dangerous cases were not picked up by the very process designed to identify and protect them. The same report (ibid.: 4) notes that:

> In many cases parents were hostile to helping agencies and workers were often frightened to visit family homes. These circumstances could have a paralysing effect on practitioners, hampering their ability to reflect, make judgments, act clearly, and to follow through with referrals, assessments or plans. Apparent or

disguised cooperation from parents often prevented or delayed understanding of the severity of harm to the child and cases drifted.

Dangerousness: low probability – high consequences

First, we are talking about extreme cases, and about cases that have extreme kinds of emotional and relational impacts on the workers who deal with them. These dynamics work powerfully and corrosively against us doing the sensible, obvious thing in our communications with one another. Why? How? I tried to write about this in an article published in the *Guardian* newspaper during the week when the 'Baby Peter' crisis seemed to be at its height.

> Most people who systematically abuse children over long periods need to go on doing this. They are expelling something terrible and dangerous in themselves, and to remove their chosen victim is to dangerously threaten their equilibrium. They are indeed dedicated to disguising what is happening and to throwing investigators off the scent. They know that what they are doing is a terrible criminal transgression in others' eyes. For such abusers, the stakes surrounding discovery could not be higher.
>
> Second, though we see with clear hindsight the 'missed opportunities' and failures to intervene, in the 'here and now' of everyday practice social workers, doctors and police do not know that this is the case where child torture is occurring and being covered up. Such cases may well appear very similar to the many other cases where children are identified as at risk. Anyone who has ever had the unwelcome job of confronting a suspected child abuser will know about the fierce, aggressive denial that is often the response. The accused becomes dedicated to making the accuser feel and believe they are, literally, mad. The problem is that we cannot know whether this terrified reaction is that of someone rightly, or wrongly, accused. If we 'knew' we could, and would, act.
>
> The research evidence suggests that the most 'dangerous families' are anyway skilled at evading the attentions of specialist child protection services. This should not blind us to the tens of thousands of cases each year where children are protected because engagement between families and professionals succeeds. Arguably the system works well enough most of the time, in most cases. In a tiny minority, it does not. But as the saying goes, 'Hard cases make bad law.' These are hard cases indeed, and should not determine the fate of the system as a whole. Social workers have been persecuted in past decades for pursuing the possibility of child abuse into the realms of fantasy. Perhaps 'satanic abuse' was a fantasy (though can we be certain?) but 'organized abuse' and 'ritual abuse' is not. It happens. Workers investigating these cases are not just dealing with aggression and fear. They are working at the borders of sanity.
>
> (Cooper 2008)

Now these forces alone may not explain our failure to act preventatively in these cases, but they are the forces we most often ignore – inter/professional working and communication is more likely to break down in the context of working with people who very seriously do not want us to co-operate with one another.

There is a persuasive model of how professional 'failure' in the context of organizational systems comes about. It is called the 'Swiss cheese' model, and the idea is that gaps or holes or failures in functioning at a number of levels in the total system may need, as it were, to come into alignment in relation to a single case so that the case drops through the series of holes in the various slices of Swiss cheese. I have simply been trying to describe one important 'slice' that is often overlooked – the dangerousness of a small minority of families and the dedication they may have to preventing us doing our job of working together.

Working together – some forgotten research

Finally, I wanted to talk briefly about some valuable overlooked research into inter/professional working that might deepen our understanding of the strengths and difficulties of this endeavour. It was published in 1992 as a book called *Anxiety and the Dynamics of Collaboration* (Woodhouse and Pengelly 1992). It is a dense piece of work, describing a research project in which a whole range of professional groups who are expected to collaborate undertook case seminars which the researchers studied, looking for evidence of how professionals interrelate. In summary, what the researchers found is that professionals are very active in assigning rather fixed roles to one another, and by extension to themselves. This occurred on the basis of a kind of what is 'you' is definitely not 'me', and what is 'me' is definitely not 'you' dynamic. This was a powerful inter-psychic process in which, for example, most professionals agreed overtly or covertly that 'knowledge about infancy and child development' belonged to health visitors, and not to 'us'; or that 'authority issues' were centrally the remit of probation officers, rather than 'us'. This process was accompanied by subtle or not so subtle acts of emotional ascription and judgement – infancy might be associated with dependency and then denigrated, along with the professionals – health visitors – who had been assigned the role of 'experts' in this field. Fears about carrying 'authority issues' in the role as social worker were similarly projected onto others who were asked to 'carry' them. These aspects of professional role then become lost to the professions who disown them, while those assigned them may feel that they are both misrepresented and burdened with unwanted aspects of their colleagues' own roles.

Our biographies, our passions

Interestingly, this research by Woodhouse and Pengelly was conducted by people whose main work and training was as couple therapists. Perhaps something of what they found out about how professions treat each other is recognisable to us from our own more intimate relationships. The problem of how to work together in 'partnerships' is one linking idea; the question of how we sustain a confident (personal or professional) identity that does not depend on first offloading onto someone else the aspects of our identities we don't like so much is another; the more positive question of the passions that go to inform our identity is a third. I think a forgotten consideration in why it's hard to get people to adjust to new ways of working, and working together, is that the threat to loss of identity that this involves is, once again, not just a resistance to change, but the deep fear of loss of something we love. We all probably have a rich story to tell about why we chose the occupation we did choose. For most of us, in some sense, it may not really have been a choice – more that it chose us. At least that was how it was for me in becoming a social worker. My father was a priest, and his first job was as a curate in an outlying small church attached to Glasgow Cathedral. I believe the roots of my choice of profession are all about my relationship to my mother and father – a way of carrying on their work in a different, secular vein, a way of staying connected to them and also of differentiating. If this kind of thing is true for many of us, then no wonder that as individuals, as people, professional change is hard, something we may both embrace and resist.

In a rather associative way I've tried to explore the connections between the various layers that influence questions about inter/professional working:

- the task – the nature of the work we do;
- professionals as people;
- professionals as members of complex systems;
- the organizational forms that support or contain these systems.

I take it as read that each of these layers has its own particular associated tensions that make the task of inter/professional working both possible, and difficult. I think that our less bounded, more fluid, more flattened, networked public sector organizational forms do make new things possible, but equally pose new threats to professional identity that we must first understand if we are to have a chance of surmounting them.

Notes

1 Baby Peter Connelly was tortured to death in his home in North London at the age of 17 months. During his life, he had been seen somewhere between 50 and 70 times by health and social work professionals. The case caused intense public anger and dismay in the UK when the details became known in December 2008, and gave rise to a significant review of the child protection system in England.

2 In England, Serious Case Reviews, formerly known as Part 8 reviews, are commissioned by local child protection co-ordinating bodies in response to child deaths and serious injuries, where abuse is suspected. Their aim is to create learning from experience but they are currently mired in controversy in relation to questions of public access and agency accountability for 'failure'.

References

Bobbitt, P. (2003) *The shield of Achilles: war, peace and the course of history*, London: Penguin.

Brandon, M., Balderson, P., Warren, C., Howe, D., Gardner, R., Dodsworth, J. and Black, J. (2008) *Analysing child deaths and serious injury through abuse and neglect: what can we learn? A biennial analysis of Serious Case Reviews 2003–2005*, London: DCSF.

Commission for Social Care Inspection (CSCI) (2008) *Raising voices: views on safeguarding adults*, London: Commission for Social Care Inspection.

Cooper, A. (2008) 'Misguided vengeance', *Guardian*, 2 December 2008. Online. Available at: http://www.guardian.co.uk/commentisfree/2008/dec/02/baby-p-haringey-social-services-sackings (accessed 28 February 2011).

Department of Health and Home Office (DHHO) (2003) *The Victoria Climbié report of an inquiry by Lord Laming*, London: HMSO.

Giddens, A. (1994) *Beyond left and right*, Cambridge: Polity.

Halton, W. (2004) 'By what authority? Psychoanalytical reflections on creativity and change in relation to organizational life', in C. Huffington, D. Armstrong, W. Halton, L. Hoyle and J. Pooley (eds) *Working below the surface: the emotional life of contemporary organizations*, London: Karnac Books.

Laming, Lord (2009) *The protection of children in England: a progress report*, London: The Stationery Office.

Munro, E. (2011) *Munro review of child protection. Better frontline services to protect children*, London: Department for Education. Online. Available at: http://www.education.gov.uk/munroreview/downloads/Munrointerimreport.pdf (accessed 28 February 2011).

Reder, P. and Duncan, S. (2004) 'From Colwell to Climbié: inquiring into fatal child abuse', in N. Stanley and J. Manthorpe (eds) *The age of the inquiry*, London: Bruner Routledge.

Woodhouse, D. and Pengelly, P. (1992) *Anxiety and the dynamics of collaboration*, Aberdeen: Aberdeen University Press.

Chapter 3

Partnerships

The politics of agendas and policy implementation

Andrew Eccles

Introduction

This chapter looks at political aspects of the growth of partnership working across public services in the United Kingdom. It addresses three areas: the political and policy agendas in which partnership working has come to the fore; the dynamics of implementation, drawing on a literature which looks at the gap between the policy agenda and actual outcomes; and, finally, power relations in partnerships. Collaboration across agencies has become crucial to developing sound policy outcomes for service users, and putting users at the centre of services. But some key policy approaches to realize these aims in practice betray a poor understanding of policy formation and implementation, pushing ahead regardless with a set agenda. Further, the way in which political power is exercised in partnerships' and agencies' collaborative arrangements warrants scrutiny. We might indeed be 'all in this together' – to borrow a topical UK government exhortation – but that does not mean we have an equal say in setting the direction of change.

The politics of policy making

Policy and politics cannot easily be separated out. Policy does not develop in an ideological vacuum, despite recent attempts to move 'beyond left and right' (Giddens 1994) and employ a mantra of 'what works' as a guide to policy making. Attempting to separate policy from politics may be useful for politicians and administrators but is unhelpful for critical analysis. The notion that ideology might still shape policy has become further blurred by an almost universal turn to 'evidence-based' policy making. As McConnell (2010: 128) notes, evidence-based approaches have become something of a 'gold standard' in terms of public policy; the potential problem here, because of its appeal to rationality over ideology, is that 'evidence-based policy modernizes and depoliticizes policy making'. The ideological sleight of hand revolves around whose evidence is privileged. The notion that policy is somehow more rational because it is evidence based also supports a technicist focus on implementation without recourse to wider arguments or context. This narrow focus may be reinforced by an emphasis on policy success based primarily on the process of policy change rather than on wider outcomes, not least because process is easier to measure than outcomes. Key performance measures for the development of partnership working are a case in point. The measurement of implementational success has become a salient feature of public sector management in recent years (Kirkpatrick, Ackroyd and Walker 2005). Thus, if evaluations are essentially grouped around operational issues – 'tight grip evaluation' (McConnell 2010: 164) – there is no scope for critical engagement with the policy itself; the need for the policy becomes self-evident, beyond critique. Contracts to undertake evaluations of government policy are often very time limited, effectively precluding wider contextual analysis or in-depth inquiry. This emphasis on evidence, measurement of process and narrow, limited evaluation essentially accepts the policy makers' parameters for enquiry at the expense of more rounded intellectual engagement. Evidence and knowledge are not the same thing.

Problems in the implementation of partnership working policy could have been foreseen. A good research base indicated the specific issues that were likely to present themselves. That the recent headlong drive towards partnership working policy proceeded unreflectively without much reference to existing research suggests that a wider ideological agenda surrounding the notion of partnership was in play. Disentangling this ideological agenda from the many merits of, and need for, better collaborative practice is not a straightforward task. But at the very least we need to be aware of the wider agendas in which partnership working sits.

The development of policy around partnership working

In a very obvious sense partnership working which enhances communication and the exchange of ideas is a positive development, especially if it leads to speedier decision-making processes and more effective engagement with service users. But the idea of partnership has played a wider and more powerful role over the past decade and the reasons for this are more nuanced than just better practice outcomes.

For New Labour, the UK government from 1997–2010, partnership working became intricately tied in to a 'modernizing' agenda underpinned by a 'third way' ideology moving beyond market-based and state-based models. Thus, the notion of partnership carries ideological freight beyond organizational arrangements in public services or common agendas in service delivery; it became a policy loadstone defining the New Labour approach. Partnership became the underpinning logic of reform but also its modus operandi. Ling (2000) notes that partnership working has become a catch-all phrase; one that is so lacking in precision that analysis of its impact and outcomes also becomes difficult. This is perhaps not entirely unintentional: absence of clarity allows for claims of policy success on a post hoc basis. Nonetheless, for an organization not to be seen to be engaging in partnership working over the past decade – regardless of what the outcomes of this might be – would have been regarded as heretical.

In parallel, a powerful discourse has emerged around the impact, perceived or actual, of *poor* partnership working across agencies. Barrett, Sellman and Thomas (2005: 13) note that 'the lack of collaborative practice between agencies and professions is seen as being responsible for individual tragedies as well as for the failure to tackle general social problems such as social exclusion, homelessness, and crime and disorder'. In a prominent example, the Laming Report (DHHO 2003) into the death of Victoria Climbié, with its 108, primarily organizational, recommendations for service change, made a headline feature of the weak collaborative practice in the case, but further scrutiny of such inquiries invariably points to a more complex picture beneath the headlines. The subsequent 2009 Laming Report on the death of Peter Connelly, for example, notes that front-line staff in social work were 'overstretched', and case loads frequently 'very high' in an 'under-resourced' profession where 'front-line social workers and managers are under an immense amount of pressure' (Laming 2009: 44).Whilst better communication and collaborative understanding across agencies are of key importance, issues of communication and organization should not deflect from the context in which these failures in human services occur: complex issues around risk; work-force staffing levels and morale; and the fact that human services by definition will never be perfectible. The solutions to these issues are conceptually complex and politically difficult to address. The point here – given the discourse of collaboration over the past decade – is the risk of an unrealistic burden of expectation being placed on the partnership agenda for delivering service improvement, especially when we know that breaking down inter/professional barriers needs to be approached with some caution (for example, one profession's information sharing perhaps being another profession's breach of confidentiality). But the weight of expectation around partnership working may be of benefit to government, allowing solutions to be seen as primarily organizational and interagency responsibilities beyond further government involvement. Either this or, as Dunleavy (1995) suggests, governments may attach such unrealistic outcomes to policy that the resulting perceived policy failure ('failing' schools, for example) will be deemed to require intervention by central government allowing it to shape outcomes more directly. Whichever, when it comes to engaging in collaborative practice, the front line faces a difficult task.

Beyond the broader ideological aspirations of government, collaborative working is pursued in the difficult context of 'turbulent fields' (Hudson 1987). This is centred on three problematic issues. First, other legislative or organizational change affecting the professions might impact on their ability or willingness to collaborate. Second, the inability of agencies which are collaborating to meet demand from service users. Third, a retrenching economy. Any cursory look at the past decade would spot the plethora of policy changes affecting public services. Service user demand, almost by definition, cannot be wholly satisfied but ebbs on a tide of higher or lower ability to deliver. For over a decade we have witnessed a relatively high tide of service delivery in an economy underpinned by unprecedented year-on-year growth. Future signs are a good deal less propitious. Nonetheless, discussion about more collaborative working across agencies has not abated. In an era in which very substantial change is expected across health, education and social services, with reduced workforces, it seems reasonable to raise the idea that more generic, and not just collaborative, working in which the traditional distinctions across disciplines are loosened might also be under consideration. Questions of professional identities, professional status and professional discretion and accountability constitute barriers to collaboration at the best of times (Dalley 1989; Hudson 2002) and are likely to prove particularly problematic in a period of acute turbulence for front-line services in their ability to meet service user needs. The effects of fiscal retrenchment may drive professions to defend their identities and value bases. Alternatively, fiscal constraints may be on such a scale that debates around the finer points of professional status will become overwhelmed by the need to find strategies to cope with the sheer scale of restructuring of service delivery currently mooted, at least in England. The past decade of collaborative working may only have heralded a future of generic service delivery. If fiscal turbulence is most likely to be felt in social services, organizational turbulence is also more likely as a result of the current UK Conservative–Liberal coalition government changes to primary health care in England, with the proposal for a much more competitive culture. This may cut across existing partnership arrangements even within health care itself. Changes in health care, and in other areas (for example, in education with the introduction of 'free' schools), are not being replicated in other UK polities and so may serve as a fascinating comparative laboratory for the study of the effects of radical social policy change. Current organizational arrangements in Scotland appear to have created a more conducive climate for partnership working than in England, while the future for partnership working in the more fragmented landscape of radical change that seems to be developing in England is less clear.

Does partnership working make a difference?

Whether or not partnerships actually make a difference to policy outcomes raises a new set of issues to consider. In the absence of a clear understanding of the terms of reference of partnership working, what needs to be evaluated? Given the complexities of the policy context that surrounds partnerships, how far should evaluation embrace the wider policy sphere or be limited to process and organizational arrangements (Balloch and Taylor 2001)? The salience of partnership working to the political project of New Labour and the importance of policy being *seen* to be successful (Jenkins 2007), which has become indistinguishable from the success (however measured) of *actual* policy outcomes, means that we might approach the methodologies of evaluation with a more critical gaze. Cameron and Lart (2003: 15) in their review of partnership working point out that 'very few of the studies looked at either the prior question of why joint work should be seen as a "good thing" and therefore why it should be done, or at the subsequent question of what difference joint working made'. Outcomes measurement in human services is complex in any case. Outcomes measurement across agencies introduces a whole host of variables which are not easy to control, or measure (El Ansari, Phillips and Hammick 2001). Given the complexity of the variables involved, how can we know that changes in outcomes have been influenced specifically by new collaborative arrangements? This is why actual evaluations of partnership working have tended to concentrate on arrangements for partnership and the processes of their subsequent development (Dowling, Powell and Glendinning 2004). As Heenan and Birrell (2006: 64) note, 'the unrelenting drive towards the integration of health and social care in Britain has been largely politically driven with scant evidence to support the view that it will result in significant improvements'.

Moreover, the methodologies of measuring success in outcomes might attract scepticism across different agencies. Social workers, for example, would argue that quantitative methods are clearly limited in their capacity to evaluate human services. But beyond the question of methodology lies the further query of what *constitutes* a good outcome and whether its merits are similarly perceived across agencies. It has taken several years for the emphasis in partnership evaluation to move from process to outcomes for service users and for more innovative ways of looking at evaluation to be considered (Dickinson 2009) but the difficulties of attributing outcomes to partnership working remain. Indeed, such is the overall weakness of evidence to link organizational arrangements to outcomes that more recent research by Perkins *et al.* has argued that:

> Given the continuing appeal of partnerships, and their pervasiveness in all sectors of public policy, two questions arise: (1) how long is it necessary or acceptable to wait in order to be able to establish whether partnerships are having any tangible effects? And (2): would it not make more sense, and be in the spirit of 'evidence-based policy', to begin to look elsewhere for solutions?
>
> (Perkins *et al.* 2010: 113)

An additional difficulty in evaluation lies in the question of attribution – who is responsible for the success or otherwise of policy outcomes? In an ideal world of partnership working this question would not matter, as there would be collective ownership of the successes or failures. But the organizations that policy exhorts to engage in collaboration have been subject to a much more competitive policy agenda in recent years (for example, league tables across agencies, or hospital star ratings). Performance indicators to assess outcomes comparatively *within* sectors are not readily useful across different sectors. Organizations have become geared to meeting internal targets to meet the needs of sectoral analysis. In a target-driven performance culture, meeting the targets is a key concern. Where are the targets carrying similar weight which consider strategic thinking and measure outcomes across different agencies in the broader picture of service delivery? The period of New Labour and the previous Conservative administrations of the 1980s and 1990s have seen organizations retreat inwards in the face of intrusive levels of inspection, audit and performance targets (see Miller 2005 for an illuminating discussion). Thus, the climate in which partnership working has been expected to take hold has not been conducive to particularly creative or open thinking. Nor is the immediate future upbeat: it will take time for the audit and performance-indicator mindset in public agencies to relax, as there is substantial vested interest for those engaged in the target and inspection culture – the bureaucracies created to patrol the bureaucracies – to maintain the process.

Where evaluations have centred on measuring the outcomes of collaborative practice the complexity of disentangling evaluation variables becomes evident. Brown, Tucker and Domokos (2003) looked at the service outcomes for older people who were variously subject to delivery based on integrated teams and separate disciplines. There were no significant differences between the two approaches. But the variables involved and the unpredictability of changes in well-being amongst the recipients on integrated service delivery make it particularly difficult to measure the impact of the integrated approach per se. Some qualitative measures – for example on how staff in different agencies experience integrated working – might give better insight. Research reporting the experiences of front-line staff in collaborative settings do exist (Molyneux 2001) but need to contend with a dominant paradigm in organizations themselves of 'measuring the measurable' and a performance indicator culture of inquiry. Clearly, use of such qualitative approaches would have to be accepted as valid by the different professions under evaluation, but some risks are now needed to innovate evaluation techniques beyond the primary concern of organizations with fulfilling discipline-specific performance indicators or recording only development in partnership processes. Or indeed, as Perkins *et al.* (2010: 113) suggest, it may be time to 'look elsewhere for solutions'.

Arguably, partnership working has been better developed in Scotland than in England (Hudson 2007; Petch 2008). Two issues in particular might explain this. First, Scotland's public services – in particular, health – have been subject to less competitive organizational change than in England (Kerr cited in Hudson 2007: 4). Second, the drive towards partnership working was pursued in a more top-down fashion in England with a strong element of 'mandated collaboration' (Clarke and Glendinning 2002). Scotland's approach saw more detailed policy scrutiny in the post-devolution Scottish Parliament committee system (albeit that the subsequent circulars and directives remained prescriptive and mandatory). Thus, the different political and social policy arrangements in Scotland appear to have impacted on the capacity for development of collaborative working. But despite the more fertile policy terrain in Scotland for collaboration there remain obstacles to productive collaborative working. For example, the reorganization of local government in Scotland in 1996 produced a weak organizational model for collaboration with other agencies and, indeed, sustainability of essential services. The institution of the Scottish Parliament in 1999 created a further tension, this time between centre and locality. The whole question of local government responsibility for community care – the service area which has been at the forefront of partnership arguments following publication of *Modernising Community Care* (SO 1998) – has come under scrutiny, with the suggestion that it be delivered more from the centre, given the fragmentation of current organizational arrangements (Gallagher, Gibb and Mills 2007). In this sense the organizational arrangements – even in the small polity of Scotland – are flawed both vertically between the centre and locality and horizontally across the incongruent territorial boundaries of agencies. The spatial arrangements of local government have recently been subject to discussion among politicians with the suggestion that a return to the kind of larger regional clusters that pre-dated local government reorganization may be necessary for service delivery both to function effectively and to achieve some economies of scale. More recently – and more radically – there are proposals for unitary services (police, health and social care) delivered no longer at local but at national, Scottish, level. Thus, partnership working has had to contend with the sub-optimal legacy of local government arrangements that were devised for particular political agendas (territorial advantage, attacking power bases) and without devolution on the landscape. But devising new, more centralized, arrangements asks important questions about transparency, accountability and sensitivity to the democratic process. The contrast here with the radical devolution of decision-making in England (viz.

general practitioners as NHS fundholders and 'free' schools taken out of local authority control) is stark. Each system will present its own set of challenges to inter/professional working. If we add to these agendas an overriding policy thrust across the United Kingdom, of the 'personalization' and 'individualization' agenda, particularly in community care services, strategic collaborative working faces constant, externally-driven obstacles to negotiate.

The politics of implementation

Much has previously been written about the 'implementation gap' (Pressman and Wildavsky 1973) between policy making and actual delivery, the need to view policy and implementation as a continuum rather than discrete stages, and the importance of front-line professionals being afforded discretion in decision-making (Lipsky 1980; Barrett and Fudge 1981; Evans and Harris 2004; Bergen 2005). There is a tension here. Implementation which is enacted along the express designs of policy makers risks being unworkable as tactical discretion, local knowledge and the ability to adapt to changing circumstances are likely to be better handled by front-line professionals. But this level of implementational discretion risks the policy being submerged under professional vested interests and bureaucratic inertia. A further problem with policy implementation around partnership working is the different governance arrangements of the various partners involved. For example, social services departments are subject to local democratic mandate through local government. Health services are not. This may lead to multiple approaches to local implementation. Using Scotland as an example, one of the first products of partnership thinking in community care was the notion of a shared assessment tool across different agencies. But different assessment tools were introduced in neighbouring local authorities even though they might geographically sit within the same health board area. Other central–local tensions can get played out in this implementation stage: given the population of Scotland (effectively only half of metropolitan London) and the diminution of local government power in recent years to the point of homogeneity, there is a logic in centralizing service delivery (Gallagher, Gibb and Mills 2007). But this is also precisely why local authorities might strive to retain different approaches – as part of a struggle to maintain their political identity. That adjacent areas are subject to different types of service delivery is about democratic decision-making and local ownership of policy, but may be electorally threatening to government at the centre given the territorial scale involved. This threat to the centre is often presented under the rubric of a need to address 'postcode lotteries' in local service delivery, but its solution is potentially a threat to local decision-making.

Aside from spatial arrangements, another prerequisite for successful policy implementation is adequate time to carry through policy change. Public policy is littered with initiatives which needed time to bed in but were rarely afforded it. Partnership working is a particularly complex issue in which to expect rapid progress. The need for flexibility, speed of change in patterns of delivery, and attitudinal shifts in organizations with long-standing, discrete working cultures is challenging. In this respect the implementation of partnership working was flawed through overly ambitious timetables. This left partnership organizations in the position of agreeing protocols without a detailed sense of how these would be implemented in practice, with operational managers struggling to deliver. Work on joint training and developing an understanding of different working cultures took second place to process. Deficiencies in information sharing systems meant that there were often additional burdens on staff time, creating friction between some staff across disciplines from the outset. As El Ansari and Phillips (2005) note, there needs to be seen to be *demonstrable* benefits for front-line staff engaged in partnership working for the project to take root. A further aspect of implementation which might impact on the success of policy is the common use and understanding of language. Again, the different approaches to conceptualizing issues impacting on service users across professions is well documented (Dalley 1989) and there is some evidence from the early evaluations of joint working that professionals are apt to retreat into their own enclaves when faced with this unfamiliarity.

Two further aspects of the implementation process are worth noting here. First, as previously noted, there have been excellent examples of inter/professional working. The particular qualities underlying this are complex, but the willingness of individuals to engage across boundaries is a clear factor. As a systematic approach this falls short (relying largely on key personnel to make universal processes work is at best unpredictable). But it remains the case that some staff are more disposed to collaborative working than others and the level of contribution may vary across different tasks. This is not always about resistance or latter-day Luddism; Cooper (q.v.) deftly explores the underlying reasons why staff are attracted to working in particular professions in the first instance, with the result that they may be more or less willing to work outside the boundaries of certain value bases. Policy advocates and 'change managers' might well imagine that the inter/professional tasks they envisage being undertaken offer no threat to these value bases, but this is not necessarily a view shared by front-line staff. A reading of Bourdieu's notion of 'habitus' (Hillier and Rooksby 2002; and see Garrett 2007 for a useful discussion) and the way in which professional disciplines not only shape their world but develop 'durable dispositions' based on their history, training and practices might play a useful role here for those charged with driving change. As Brubaker notes:

> it is the habitus that determines the kinds of problems that are posed, the kinds of instruments (conceptual, methodological, statistical) that are employed. Most important, the habitus determines the manner in which problems are posed, explanations constructed, and instruments employed.
>
> (Brubaker in Garrett 2007: 358)

Thus, it is not necessarily that professions are unwilling to engage with others; it is that the sense they make of a given situation will be constrained by their unconscious understanding of the world developed through their history and practice. The attempt to cross disciplinary barriers is not a straightforward, 'quick fix' task; this explains why process and organizationally driven reforms are unlikely to succeed in crossing deeply embedded discipline-based outlooks.

Second, where there has been good inter/professional working the organizational arrangements have often been ad hoc or informal. It is the formalization of arrangements, sometimes initiated by these same change managers, which may undermine good working procedures that have developed more organically over time. None of this understanding about the complexities and difficulties of implementation is an argument against collaborative working. Much of it, however, offers cautionary guidance about a reliance on overly rigid structures. Looser arrangements may work better, as more recent work examining networks in Scottish health and social care arrangements would suggest (Hudson 2007).

Returning to the site where the recent push towards collaborative practice has worked better, there are two aspects of the Scottish polity which operate in favour of successful implementation of partnership working. First, the areas at the core of the collaborative working agenda, initially social care and health, followed by education, are the key departmental responsibilities of the devolved Scottish polity and thus initiatives in this area carry particular political weight. Equally, the flagship policy that distinguished the new Scottish Parliament in its early days was implementation of the recommendations of the *Sutherland Report* (Royal Commission on Long Term Care 1999) in favour of free personal care for older people. Part of the rationale for free personal care as argued by Sutherland was that it represented a way of bridging the historic budgetary and organizational divide between health and social care over service provision; in other words, that it might facilitate easier working across agencies. The second advantage to partnership working in Scotland was, as already noted, its less fragmented health care system. If partnership working was viable it ought to have had a better chance of succeeding in Scotland than south of the border. That it remains problematic is salutary for decision-makers in Scotland and elsewhere.

The politics of everyday working across professions

The complexities of evaluating the outcomes of partnership working have already been noted, as has the predominance of evaluations based on examining structural arrangements and processes. That notwithstanding, there is a developing literature which has started to examine the detail of how front-line staff have responded to the partnership agenda. In this sense – outcomes aside – there is now evidence of the practice of partnership working within these structures and processes (Tett, Crowther and O'Hara 2003; McNamara 2006; Eccles 2008). These studies resonate with the difficulties of policy implementation that have been discussed above and illustrate the micropolitics of everyday working: issues such as workload equity, challenges to identity and access to resources. The research on collaborative working between health and social care in particular has several recurring themes. These include the predominance of training in collaborative processes but not in the further understanding of working cultures, the equity of workloads across disciplines, the different approaches to understanding ways of working with service users (for example over the issue of consent and the importance of service user narrative), and assessment of needs. These accounts of the practices of partnership working emphasize the essentially procedural way in which collaboration has been implemented: through the creation of protocols; the alignment of budgets across agencies; and statements of commitment to the partnership agenda. In part this reflects a genuine attempt by organizations to work together but there is also an element here of organizations simply responding to the demands and tight timetables set by central government. It is in managing the day-to-day operation of collaborative working that the problems arise, with inconsistent commitment by middle managers to achieving the outcomes required the often aspirational rubric of partnership protocols.

Stewart, Petch and Curtice (2003) discuss some of the operational drivers and barriers to partnership working, noting the barriers that might be put in place through resistance to change by professionals unreflectively adhering to existing patterns of working. But equally some resistance may arise from situations where professionals are concerned about how collaboration might impact adversely on the experience of service users. This takes the discussion beyond simply the processes of better working through collaboration (which might deal with, for example, eliminating unnecessary duplication of assessments by different agencies) into territory which deals with value bases or inadequate grounding in an understanding of different working cultures in the new collaborative process itself (Dalley 1989; Hudson 2002). Thus, for example, assessment frameworks devised to reduce duplication of assessments by different health and social care agencies have been inconsistently utilized by staff (Eccles 2008). The assessment tool was designed to be handled with equal ease across professional disciplines but front-line staff noted discrepancies in its use, most particularly in areas such as personal narrative or detail about service users' sources of income. This raises a clear dilemma: not duplicating service user assessments may improve efficiency but if the quality of assessment is lessened in the process does this necessarily constitute a gain for the service user? As initial service user assessments can lack consistency of approach, there might be grounds for wariness here about further expansion of more generic approaches. Recent research on shared assessment frameworks used across children's services involving social services, health and education (Aldgate 2011) offers a very varied picture of their impact in different settings across the UK. Aldgate argues that where there has been a less prescriptive approach and more local ownership of frameworks and their specific local implementation, as in Scotland, early results have been positive (see also MacNeil and Stradling 2010, who note better quality and consistency of information). Nevertheless, a key issue about assessment frameworks remains, that is, what is the conceptual or value base on which assessment frameworks build (Crisp *et al.* 2007)? Are shared assessment frameworks perceived similarly across professions? What elements that are viewed as important to particular professions might be compromised in the pursuit of shareable information or organizational neatness?

Organizational arrangements and assessment frameworks cannot readily be isolated from resource issues. Prioritization of resources in service delivery remains a key issue. Rationing of the allocation of services takes place across the different agencies. For social workers this is explicit: assessments are made on the basis of need (although assessors know in advance that all needs cannot be met). These needs will then be prioritized. This process of rationing is likely to be less transparent in health care. Part of the move towards more inter/professional working has seen staff from different professional backgrounds designated as key workers whose role is to be the individual most responsible for subsequent engagement with service users. This has had the considerable merit of simplifying points of contact for service users. It has also introduced health staff more clearly to the politics of rationing and a world of uncertainty over service delivery. Assessment for service users may be made more quickly using a single process but those who have been assessed may then effectively still sit in a system where service delivery is prioritized, particularly if its funding is based on a social services budget. This can cause unease for workers with different professional experiences around translating needs into delivery in different settings.

Partnerships and power relations

In this section the significance of power differentials among the different partners is examined, particularly issues of variable accountability, democratic access and political clout. Historically, medicine – and to some extent education – can lay claim to having been particularly influential professions in policy making (albeit unevenly depending on prevailing political priorities) based on their expert knowledge and position of political importance in the public domain (Jordan and Richardson 1987). Social work has rarely enjoyed similar influence or professional standing and until recently has been viewed as a semi-profession (Toren 1972). Thus, beneath partnership protocols, long-standing differences in power remain. Research into health and social services collaboration (Wilkin, Gillam and Leese 2000) noted some very clear distinctions about which voice – predominantly, health – was more likely to influence the agenda where there are joint arrangements. Where there have been long-established organizational collaborations – for example, in Northern Ireland – the health agenda will tend to emerge as more powerful in practice (Heenan and Birrell 2006).

The power of 'agenda setting' in organizations (Lukes 2005) is an issue that would benefit from more enquiry in the current partnership policy drive. Since the exercise of power is not always observable, agenda setting assumes greater importance given the introduction in some localities of single management structures across health and social care (such as Community Health Care Partnerships in Scotland) as a response to the problems of joint working arrangements that had been overseen by bifurcated management structures. On the face of it, a plurality of ideas coming from health and social care which feed into a common agenda is a welcome development, but whosoever holds sway within the organization exercises power (Schattscheider, in Lukes 2005: 71). As noted, the exercise of this power is not necessarily obvious. Single management structures offer the possibility for a plurality of issues about health and social need to be tabled, but they equally have the potential for a medical agenda, based on a historic balance of power, to subsume the debate. Thus there may be a plurality of input from different professions, but who might set the agenda and prevail in the decision-making still needs to be understood.

On a broader issue these new partnership structures sit as part of governance arrangements that have seen local government increasingly operate as part of a wider network of agencies, which have (often significantly) more indirect democratic accountability, altering the politics of representation. Writing about local politics,

Wolman and Goldsmith (1992) viewed local government as an 'arena of well-being', but essential aspects of this well-being – such as housing services, and increasingly education and an array of arm's length agencies – may now lie outside local authority control and sit instead in the wider local partnership frameworks with their new forms of accountability. This increasingly complex array of governance arrangements, with its attendant blurred lines of accountability and transparency, may accommodate the semblance of partnership working but simultaneously lack clear lines of accessibility and obscure very real professional tensions. With its budgetary divisions and sectoral performance management, recent public policy itself emerges, in part, as antithetical to the kind of clarity needed to inform partnership working. Public policy which impacts on the issue of partnerships has been pulling in different directions; while each direction has its own internal political logic, the total effect is to weaken the likelihood of collaborative success.

There are strong resonances here, in the pervasive incidence of the use of the term partnership, with the notion of 'community', particularly as it has been used in relation to community care over the past fifteen years. There is a substantial literature (see for example Symonds and Kelly 1998) which draws out the imprecision of meaning in community; is community a territorial designation or an expression of a community of interests? Can it be both, given the inherent tensions between the two, and in what ways is community understood by different professional disciplines, carers or service users? How can we reconcile the use of community as an adjunct to care when communities themselves can be exclusionary or judgemental (Bauman 2001)? Community clearly has some seductive overtones. With its essentially positive implications, and despite its imprecision as a term, who could argue against it? Yet under the rubric of 'community care' profound changes to the organization of services and a reshaping of the role of public bodies and their relationship to the independent sector took place. So too with partnership: the term embodies a central plank of a policy discourse which has tried to square public services within the circle of a continuing market-driven agenda, but leaves in its wake a raft of imprecision over power relations, value bases and working practices. That forms of partnership working seem better placed to work in Scotland says something about a more distinctive (and perhaps in parts still collectivist) Scottish policy identity within the UK. But even here there is still a need to disentangle the various layers of political power and organizational structures that simultaneously promote and in practice may detract from the partnership agenda. Here, also, limits to partnership working may have been seen with the demise of the largest of Scotland's Community Health Care Partnerships – the single management structure umbrella organization for primary health and social care – after some four years of operation (Braiden 2011). This will be remembered, in part, by front-line workers and operational managers for the effort expended in creating and participating in the partnership arrangement; effort which might better have been focused on smaller-scale, less ambitious, locally based collaborative practice with more recognizable – and perhaps measurable – impact. As it stands, the recriminations around the end of the partnership suggest it may have been a move too far, too soon.

Partnership working through technological capacity

So far it has been argued that the move towards partnership working across agencies has been predominantly process driven; that is, through working arrangements, management structures or shared assessment tools. The drive to push on with integrated working is now informed by increased technological capacity. Thus one of the perceived weaknesses of collaborative working arrangements – the absence of information technology adequate to the task – is no longer viewed as such an impediment. In children's services, the use of technology has been most apparent in data gathering and sharing, with a particularly high profile example being the Integrated Children's System deployed in statutory children's social care. Here, the technological capacity has, in itself, partly driven the shape and pace of change in integrated working, most especially in England. This has also proved problematic. A study of the Integrated Children's System by White *et al.* (2010) reveals a catalogue of systemic failure in design and implementation which, they argue, has impacted adversely on the ability of front-line workers to operate with adequate professional discretion. That these failures were predictable (and were, indeed, predicted) was lost in an overriding desire of government to 'modernize' services and introduce models of information sharing software wholly unsuitable for the needs of human services. The process also revealed a familiar top-down model of implementation brought to bear on local authorities by the Department of Children, Schools and Families which resisted informed critique by local authorities about the shortcomings of the system. White *et al.* (ibid.: 410, brackets added) note that: 'All [respondents] were negative, not necessarily about the idea and the aspirations associated with electronic recording, in which many could see great potential; rather the contours of this particular model were ubiquitously a source of immense frustration. . . .' Part of the problem here is the need to make information fit into particular categories for the purposes of recording. Devising systems that require data recording across different agencies has the potential to exacerbate the loss of nuance in a bid for a shared data set. Such process-driven approaches, which too rapidly developed into collaborative arrangements that were weak in interagency understandings of role and value base, are likely now to have a technology-driven logic which will allow the accretion of more information and the capacity for its dissemination across agencies. This – given the experience of the Integrated Children's System agency – begs significant questions about the utility of processes and quality of information. The problem here lies, in part, around the nature of human services themselves and the prevalence of complexity in human services' decision-making. This is the territory of 'wicked issues': issues that are complex, that do not have formulaic solutions and that are not likely to be replicated in very predictable patterns (Hudson and Henwood 2002). There are no straightforward solutions based on large-scale structural reform, neither of organizational arrangements nor information systems and particularly not of the kind that the 'modernization' of public services have spawned in recent years. White *et al.* (2010) and Eccles (2008) both note a clear willingness on the part of front-line workers to be part of these changes; it is primarily the process-driven nature of reforms that arouses staff hostility and so the terms on which collaboration and information sharing across agencies takes place need to be rethought to avoid frustration becoming all too synonymous with attempts at integrated or collaborative working.

Conclusion

A number of political issues have emerged here. There are tensions around partnership working which take in questions of governance and organization across agencies, relationships between centre and locality, and where precisely partnerships sit as part of wider, more ideologically-driven agendas. At a more micro level, differentials in power across professions have strong historical roots, while the professions themselves tend to have long-held value bases. In an era of evidence-based policy change there is a singular lack of clear evidence that the arrangements put in place over the past decade have impacted significantly on outcomes. There are anecdotal accounts of successful collaborative working, but these often seem to be contingent on local circumstances and shared ideas. This suggests that the overly 'top-down' approach to managing partnership working has in itself proved problematic.

Some of the political tensions on display are about a resistance to change (or, as the rubric would have it, a failure to 'modernize'). But this modernization agenda is based on some powerful ideological, and not just practical, underpinnings that raise questions about the wider direction of public services. In this sense the resistance to change may be in response to the underlying modernization agenda itself rather than partnerships per se. Thus, partnership working sits in the middle of this complex mix – meeting the needs of the public but also subject to wider political complexities, including a performance-indicator culture, that may be inimical to better collaboration. What is needed now is less evidence from narrowly focused evaluations and an appeal instead to our knowledge and understanding of how organizations work best together. This should include some scepticism about attempts to depoliticize policy implementation and evaluation and instead appreciate the need to work with the grain of the political dynamics involved in policy change.

References

Aldgate, J. (2011) 'Ensuring that every child really does matter', in M. Hill, F. McNeil and R. Taylor (eds) *21st Century social workers: a resource for early professional development*, London: BASW/Venture Press.

Balloch, S. and Taylor, M. (2001) (eds) *Partnership working. Policy and practice*, Bristol: The Policy Press.

Barrett, S. and Fudge, C. (1981) (eds) *Policy and action: essays on the implementation of public policy*, London: Methuen.

Barrett, G., Sellman, D. and Thomas, J. (2005) *Interprofessional working in health and social care*, Basingstoke: Palgrave.

Bauman, Z. (2001) *Community: seeking safety in an insecure world*, Cambridge: Cambridge University Press.

Bergen, A. (2005) '"Implementation deficit" and "street level bureaucracy": policy practice and change in the development of community nursing issues', *Health and Social Care in the Community* 13: 1–10.

Braiden, G. (2011) 'Health board breaks up key partnerships', *The Herald*, 19 May. Online. Available at: http://www.heraldscotland.com/news/health/health-board-breaks-up-key-partnerships-1.1028779 (accessed 26 March 2011).

Brown, L., Tucker, C. and Domokos, T. (2003) 'Evaluating the impact of integrated health and social care teams on older people living in the community', *Health and Social Care in the Community* 11: 85–94.

Cameron, A. and Lart, R. (2003) 'Factors promoting and obstacles hindering joint working: a systematic review of the research evidence', *Journal of Integrated Care* 11: 9–17.

Clarke, C. and Glendinning, C. (2002) 'Partnership and the remaking of welfare governance', in C. Glendinning, M. Powell and K. Rummery (eds) *Partnerships, New Labour and the governance of welfare*, Bristol: Policy Press.

Crisp, B., Anderson, M., Orme, J. and Green Lister, P. (2007) 'Assessment frameworks: a critical reflection', *British Journal of Social Work* 37: 1059–77.

Dalley, G. (1989) 'Professional ideology or organizational tribalism? The health service–social work divide', in R. Taylor and J. Ford (eds) *Social work and health care*, London: Jessica Kingsley.

Department of Health and Home Office (DHHO) (2003) *The Victoria Climbié Report of an Inquiry by Lord Laming*, London: HMSO.

Dickinson, H. (2009) 'The outcomes of health and social care partnerships', in J. Galsby and H. Dickinson (eds) *International perspectives on health and social care*, Oxford: Blackwell.

Dowling, B., Powell, M. and Glendinning, C. (2004) 'Conceptualising successful partnerships', *Health and Social Care in the Community* 12: 309–17.

Dunleavy, P. (1995) 'Policy disasters: explaining the UK's record', *Public Policy and Administration* 10: 52–70.

Eccles, A. (2008) 'Single shared assessment: the limits to "quick fix" implementation', *Journal of Interprofessional Care* 16: 22–30.

El Ansari, W. and Phillips, C. (2005) 'The costs and benefits to participants in community partnerships: a paradox?' *Health Promotion Practice* 5: 35–48.

El Ansari, W., Phillips, C. J. and Hammick, M. (2001) 'Collaboration and partnerships: developing the evidence base', *Health and Social Care in the Community* 9: 215–27.

Evans, T. and Harris, J. (2004) 'Street level social work, bureaucracy and the (exaggerated) death of discretion', *British Journal of Social Work* 34: 871–95.

Gallagher, J., Gibb, K. and Mills, C. (2007) 'Rethinking central local government relations in Scotland: back to the future?', *Hume Occasional Paper* 70, Glasgow: David Hume Institute/University of Glasgow.

Garrett, P. M. (2007) 'The relevance of Bourdieu for social work', *Journal of Social Work* 7: 355–79.

Giddens, A. (1994) *Beyond left and right – the future of radical politics*, Cambridge: Polity Press.

Heenan, D. and Birrell, D. (2006) 'The integration of health and social care: the lessons from Northern Ireland', *Social Policy and Administration* 40: 47–66.

Hillier, J. and Rooksby, E. (eds) (2002) *Habitus: a sense of place*, Aldershot: Ashgate.

Hudson, B. (1987) 'Collaboration in welfare: a framework for analysis', *Policy and Politics* 15: 175–82.

—— (2002) 'Inter-professionality in health and social care: the Achilles' heel of partnership?', *Journal of Inter-Professional Care* 16: 7–18.

—— (2007) 'Partnering through networks: can Scotland crack it?', *Journal of Integrated Care* 15: 3–13.

Hudson, B. and Henwood, M. (2002) 'The NHS and social care: the final countdown?', *Policy and Politics* 30: 153–66.

Jenkins, R. (2007) 'The meaning of policy/policy as meaning', in S. Hodgson and Z. Irving (eds) *Policy reconsidered*, Bristol: Policy Press.

Jordan, A. G. and Richardson, J. (1987) *Government and pressure groups in Britain*, Oxford: Clarendon Press.

Kirkpatrick, I., Ackroyd, S. and Walker, R. (2005) *The new managerialism and public service professions*, Basingstoke: Palgrave Macmillan.

Laming, Lord (2009) *The protection of children in England: a progress report*, London: The Stationery Office.

Ling, T. (2000) 'Unpacking partnership: the case of health care', in C. Clarke, S. Gewirtz and E. McLaughlin (eds) *New managerialism, new welfare?* London: Sage.

Lipsky, M. (1980) *Street level bureaucracy*, New York: Russell Sage Foundation.

Lukes, S. (2005) *Power: a radical view* (2nd edition), Basingstoke: Palgrave Macmillan.

MacNeil, M. and Stradling, B. (2010) *Getting it right for every child, briefing 6: green shoots of progress*, Edinburgh: The Scottish Government.

McConnell, A. (2010) *Understanding policy success*, Basingstoke: Palgrave.

McNamara, G. (2006) 'Implementation of single shared assessment in Meadowbank, Falkirk: a joint future', *Journal of Integrated Care* 14: 38–44.

Miller, D. (2005) 'What is best "value"? Bureaucracy, virtualism and local governance', in P. Du Gay (ed.) *The values of bureaucracy*, Oxford: Oxford University Press.

Molyneux, J. (2001) 'Interprofessional team working: what makes teams work well?', *Journal of Interprofessional Care* 15: 29–35.

Parsons, W. (1995) *Public policy*, Aldershot: Edward Elgar.

Perkins, N., Smith, K., Hunter, D. J., Bambra, C. and Joyce, K. (2010) 'What counts is "what works"? New Labour and partnerships in public health', *Policy and Politics* 38: 101–17.

Petch, A. (2008) 'Delivering health and social care: do partnerships deliver for users and carers?' Online. Available as audio at http://www.iriss.ac.uk/search/node/petch (accessed 8 March 2011).

Pressman, J. and Wildavsky, A. (1973) *Implementation. How great expectations in Washington are dashed in Oakland*, Berkley, CA: University of California Press.

Royal Commission on Long Term Care (1999) *With respect to old age: long term care: rights and responsibilities, (Sutherland Report)*, London: Stationery Office.

Scottish Office (SO) (1998) *Modernising community care*, London: HMSO.

Stewart A., Petch A. and Curtice, L. (2003) 'Moving towards integrated working in health and social care in Scotland: from maze to matrix', *Journal of Interprofessional Care* 17: 335–50.

Symonds, A. and Kelly, A. (1998) *The social construction of community care*, Basingstoke: Palgrave.

Tett, L., Crowther, J. and O'Hara, P. (2003) 'Collaborative partnerships in community education', *Journal of Education Policy* 18: 37–51.

Toren, N. (1972) *Social work: the case of a semi-profession*, Beverly Hills, CA: Sage.

White, S., Wastell, D., Broadhurst, K. and Hall, C. (2010) 'When policy o'erleaps itself: the tragic tale of the Integrated Children's System', *Critical Social Policy* 30: 405–29.

Wilkin, D., Gillam, S. and Leese, B. (2000) *The national tracker survey of primary care groups and trusts*, London: King's Fund.

Wolman, H. and Goldsmith, M. (1992) *Urban politics and policy*, Oxford: Blackwell.

Chapter 4

Transprofessional social capital in children's services
Dis/connects in policy and practice

Joan Forbes

Introduction

A key aim in education and social policy trajectories in the United Kingdom countries and other places is that all the available knowledge and skills resources of children's public sector agencies should be harnessed and applied in practice to the benefit of children and families (Forbes and Watson 2009). However, a recent study in Scotland into partnership working between education and allied health professions concluded that 'guidance is needed because many parents and practitioners are saying there is room for improvement in partnership working between allied health professionals and education staff' (SG 2010: 4). The Scottish Government report goes on to remind readers that 'this message is also clear in the HMIE report on the implementation of the Education (Additional Support for Learning) (Scotland) Act 2004' (ibid., and quoting HMIE 2007). To explore and better understand the specific forms of practitioner relations envisaged in different education and social policy trajectories, and some of the disconnects which guidance and professional codes produce in practice, this chapter draws on the concept of social capital (Coleman 1990; Bourdieu 1993; Putnam 1993) which Halpern (2005: 4) defines as, 'social networks and the norms and sanctions that govern their character. It is valued for its potential to facilitate individual and community action, especially through their solution of collective action problems.'

The current moment of children's public sector *integration* has been described as a 'paradigm shift' (Grek, Ozga and Lawn 2009) from the preceding period characterized by *inter*/professional and *inter*agency working (Hartley 2009). Integration cuts across governance, practices and knowledge bases of children's services and agencies, and concepts are needed to analyse the ways these cross-cutting trajectories operate – or conversely, do not. The following analytical distinctions are relevant here (Percy-Smith 2005: 24–5):

> **holistic government or governance** – integration and coordination at all levels and in relation to all aspects of policy-related activity – policy making, regulation, service provision and scrutiny;
>
> **cross-boundary working** – agencies working together on areas that extend beyond the scope of any one agency;

cross-cutting – issues that are not the 'property' of a single organization or agency – e.g., social inclusion, improving health;

integration – agencies working together in a single, often new, organizational structure.

This chapter examines connections which productively or otherwise cut across the work of children's sector agencies and so, at this point, the following working definitions of the key terms used here to conceptualize practitioner and agency cross-cutting relations may be helpful to the reader (cf. Brown and White 2006):

- **transprofessional** – work across professional groups on cross-cutting remits or responsibilities;
- **transdisciplinary** – work across subject disciplinary groups on cross-cutting issues, agendas or remits;
- **trans-sectoral** – a) work across two or more public sectors (e.g., education, health, social work) on cross-cutting issues; b) work across the children's and adult public sectors on cross-cutting issues.

A conceptual framework is needed which grasps such cross-cutting relations and so the frame of social capital is used here to identify and analyse the transprofessional, transdisciplinary and trans-sectoral practice relations envisaged in governance and policy. But first, recent key trajectories in policy are discussed.

Governance and policy

Globally, education and social policy is redesigning children's public services (Forbes and Watson 2009). For example, recent policy in England (the Children Act 2004, usually referred to as the *Every Child Matters* agenda; DfES 2004, 2005; DCSF 2008b) and in the United States (the No Child Left Behind Act of 2001, US Congress 2002) has driven integrated service agendas in relation to full-service schools and extended children's services and children's workforce remodelling agendas. Co-professional working is a mandatory, planned feature of such service provision. In England, the Teacher Development Agency (TDA 2007: 7) stipulates that teachers:

Have a commitment to collaboration and co-operative working, where appropriate.

And in Scotland the General Teaching Council (GTCS 2006: 10) advises that:

Registered teachers work co-operatively with other professionals, staff and parents.

Across the UK countries, government policy now mandates 'joined-up' working amongst public services (DE 2005; OFMDFM 2006; SEED 2006; DCSF 2008b). Such policies impact upon professionals through statements from separate UK professional registration bodies, to which practitioners must adhere in order to retain their professional registration and legitimacy to practice.

Earlier Scottish education and social policy which viewed schools as hubs for collaborative working (SO 1998) has given way to policy mandates that integrated services be provided in the spaces in which children's services are located (SE 2001; HMIE 2005; SE 2006a, 2006b; SEED 2006). For example, through the joint working of 'education, health, social work and a range of other agencies' Her Majesty's Inspectorate of Education sought a 'more integrated and holistic support service' (HMIE 2002: 9) to achieve social inclusion and raise educational standards. And the foregoing makes evident that the period between 2004 and 2006 is characterized by particularly critical intensive convergence in policy and legislation trajectories engendered by the *Getting it Right for Every Child* programme (SE 2005; SP 2006; SG 2008), an agenda driven in part by a wider Scottish government concern to implement cross-cutting policy effectively (SE 2000). Thus, a raft of policy across agencies has changed governance with the aim of strengthening and embedding integrated working in practice.

This key shift in policy constructions is clearly evident in, for example, *Improving Outcomes for Children and Young People: The Role of Schools in Delivering Integrated Children's Services*, in which the Scottish Executive Education Department (SEED 2006: 2) states that 'it no longer makes sense to think of schools separately from other agencies' and that there is now a wider integration agenda relating to the 'delivery of Integrated Children's Services' (ibid.: 2). In addition, since 2005 the institution of an integrated inspection regime for children's services in Scotland has driven holistic cross-boundary, transprofessional and trans-sectoral strategic and operational governance (HMIE 2005; SE 2006b). And since 2006 the new children's public sector paradigm shift has been reinforced by the introduction of the *eCare Framework*, a potential public service panopticon intended 'for the sharing of personal data across the Scottish public sector', which will in future be 'key to enabling practitioners to deliver better outcomes for the citizens of Scotland' (SG 2006).

Review of all relevant children's services policy is beyond the scope of this chapter and so analysis now focuses on the discourses in a key recent policy governing allied health professions (AHP) relations in practice with education in Scotland. It should be noted, however, that allied health professions such as speech and language therapy are distinct UK-wide professional bodies with separate registration which introduces a highly complex – and perhaps protectionist – governance and regulatory environment fraught with structural and cultural issues as an additional dimension of difficulty at all levels in efforts to merge children's services. In the UK, AHPs comprise: arts therapists; dieticians; occupational therapists; orthoptists; orthotists and prosthetisists; podiatrists; physiotherapists; diagnostic and therapeutic radiographers; and speech and language therapists (SG 2010). Since 2003, the UK Health Professions Council generic standards of proficiency have, for example, mandated both professional autonomy 'independence' and a 'collaborative team' approach. In 2007, the *Standards of Proficiency: Speech and Language Therapists* stated that registrant speech and language therapists must:

Understand the need to build and sustain professional relationships as both an independent practitioner and collaboratively as a member of a team.

(HPC 2007: section 1b.1)

The ability to work with others has become for children's public sector professional groups an index of professional fitness to practice. But critical disjunctures between the discourses of 'collaboration' policy, single profession registration requirements and single agency contractual governance and regulation, and wider children's social policy recommendations for integrated practice remain and continue to emerge. There are particular issues, for example, when professionals are employed by different public sector agencies. Across the United Kingdom countries, AHPs work for the National Health Service, thus they may view themselves in schools and other non-health settings as 'visiting' outside agency practitioners, whilst key recent policy guidance across the UK countries and beyond recommend that to achieve success for all children and young people improved transprofessional and trans-sectoral relationships are needed in policy, governance, leadership and practice. HMIE (2009: 24), for example, advises that 'educational establishments and services need to ensure positive relationships at all levels. They need to seek and build upon the views and evaluations of learners, parents and partner professionals.'

In England, the *Bercow Report* (DCSF 2008a), a review of services for children and young people with speech, language and communication needs, reiterated previous policy recommendations for transprofessional and trans-sectoral working by education and AHPs involved in the provision of such services, but noted high variability and a lack of equity in the provision of services:

> . . . coherent strategies for children and young people using a joint commissioning framework, shared goals and integrated service delivery were rare. Responses to the call for evidence reinforced this view.
>
> (DCSF 2008a: 52)

And recommended that:

> To support further the workforce to deliver [services to children and young people with speech, language and communication needs] we recommend professionals from across the children's and young people's workforce undertake pre-qualification training in collaborative and multidisciplinary working, alongside professionals from other backgrounds.
>
> (Ibid.: 9, Recommendation 20, brackets added)

Using the discourses of partnership rather than of integration, the recently published consultation in Scotland into the ways in which partnership between AHPs and education working may be developed, *Guidance on Partnership Working Between Allied Health Professions and Education* (SG 2010: 45), gives several examples of good practice, but concludes that: 'many of the challenges to partnership working are common across different services', and that 'there is still work to be done in order to understand fully how each other's services to young people are evolving and changing' (ibid.). The report exhorts practitioners that: 'Continuing to engage in open discussion and making the most of the relationships we have been building over recent times, will help to build on current good practice' (ibid.), and prescribes the 'key message' of: 'a commitment to evaluating where we are with regards to being effective partners ourselves . . . we can develop our interpersonal skills to better see another's perspective' (ibid.). The Scottish Government report, then, clearly takes the relational, social capital turn in its conclusions which specifically identify what is done, or left undone, between practitioners as the space both of difficulties and potential improvement of transprofessional and cross-boundary working practices.

Service integration, then, has emerged as a discrete and important strand in some, but not consistently all, policy and it is in the instances of policy and governance inconsistency or disjuncture that practice relation disconnects emerge introducing difficulties and uncertainties, with potentially detrimental effects for integrated practice in the currently complex space that cuts across and through children's services boundaries.

However, prior to the *Bercow Report* (DCSF 2008a) and the *Guidance on Partnership Working Between Allied Health Professions and Education* report (SG 2010) there has, in the UK, been limited government-sponsored investigation of the actual perspectives of AHPs working with education to inform policy, or research into the relationships that currently pertain amongst practitioners, or of how they might make the most of relationships, or put to use their inter/professional social capital resources.

Both these reports draw on illustrative examples of participants' comments gathered in the empirical data gathered in their research. This chapter utilizes those comments to illustrate the discussion below as exemplifications of professional relations. But, first, social capital theory is introduced as a potentially fruitful conceptual and analytical framework to discern co-practice *relations* and to explore the potential disjunctures in practice relations between teacher/AHP practitioners.

Applying social capital theory

A number of institutions involved in public policy formation have used social capital theory, notably the World Bank (Narayan 1999), OECD (2000) and the UK Government Performance and Innovation Unit (2002), placing different emphases on various of its characteristics. For example, Narayan (1999) places emphasis on the effects of social capital as the 'social glue' which holds society together; Baron, Field and Schuller (2000: 8) emphasize its value in 'providing access to new knowledge and resources'; whilst the Bourdieuian strand in social capital theory (1986) conceptualizes social (and other forms of) capital as a form of power in which networks and the resources which accrue to individuals from network membership are accumulated and held by social elites at the expense of others in a zero-sum equation, and so social capital 'may serve as currency' (Bourdieu 1977b: 503).

However, Coleman (1988) views stocks of social capital as not limited to the powerful, asserting that trust and reciprocity, key terms in social capital theory, constitute a resource for communities, and places emphasis on the role of social capital in building individuals' human capital. Coleman focuses on what social capital *does*: 'social capital is productive, making possible the achievement of certain ends that in its absence would not be possible' (ibid.: 96).

Like Coleman, Putnam (1995) views social capital as, on balance, a positive force in civic society. Putnam states that social capital lies in the productive functioning of networks of relationships based on shared norms and trust: 'social capital, in short refers to social connections and the attendant norms and trust' (ibid.: 664–5). For Putnam, social capital is a resource that functions at societal level underpinned by individuals' active participation in the social organization and networks of civic society (Putnam 1995, 2000). Viewed thus as focusing on the formation and operation of networks at individual, group and societal levels, and on the ways in which shared norms and trust underpin networks, social capital offers a potentially fruitful analytic to examine interpractitioner relations.

Applying social capital to the AHP/teacher relation

The theoretical framework of social capital is used here to identify points of disjuncture and disconnects in an analysis of education/AHP practice relationships. The social capital analytic derives from work in business and management studies (Field 2009), and has already been helpful in analysing the work of speech and language therapy AHPs and teachers (Forbes 2008).

Conceptualized as a multi-level matrix (Halpern 2005), social capital theory offers a methodological approach that moves between macro, meso and micro multi-systemic levels, i.e., the governance and policy, institutional and individual or personal planes. Following Putnam (2000), Halpern (2005: 10) identifies three basic components of social capital, including the form of interest here – work-based social capital – in the following terms: 'They consist of a *network*; a cluster of *norms, values and expectancies* . . . shared by group members; and *sanctions* – punishments and rewards – that help to maintain the norms and network.' Putnam describes sub-types of social capital connections as *bonding* (exclusive of others not in the group) and *bridging* (inclusive of non-group others) noting that bonding relations may be more 'inward looking and have a tendency to reinforce exclusive identities and homogenous groups', and in contrast, bridging relations are 'outward-looking and encompass people across different social cleavages' (Putnam 2000: 22).

A model of social capital may then be developed along these two axes: *components* and *sub-types* of social capital, allowing an analysis of relations and connections at three levels – the *inter-personal* level of intra-personal knowledge and skills; the *institutional and practice* level; and the *governance and policy* level. Such a conceptual mapping which highlights the intersections of different practitioners' and practitioner groups' (here teaching/AHP) bonding and bridging networks (connections) with professionals' norms and values and trust allows practitioners' inter/professional level social capital to be identified and analysed.

The themes discussed draw on empirical insights in data excerpts from *Guidance on Partnership Working Between Allied Health Professions and Education* (SG 2010).

These illustrative quotations are used to provoke lines of discussion concerning trans-professional social capital in a specific policy-practice disjuncture amongst prevailing education and allied health professions policy with built-in difficulties for integration-in-practice.

Integrating-in-practice – or not: AHP/teacher social capital

The Scottish Government (SG 2010: 12) document uses a comment attributed to 'Allied Health Professional and Teacher' to illustrate integration-in-practice:

> We can see that the child's progress has been greater than we would have expected and that we have achieved more working on this programme together than if we had been going our own ways.

Here the practitioners attest to the benefits to the child of co-practice characterized by joint problem solving in a practical support context, and knowledge and skills exchange in a relation of interpractitioner confidence and reciprocity.

In other circumstances, however, teachers may well consider – and resent – a teacher/therapist relationship consisting mainly – or solely – of delegating tasks and programmes to them in a 'traditional' teaching/AHP consultancy approach, viewing such practices as workload off-loading by a separate service practitioner. Whilst the Scottish government recognizes that:

> Some of the most important roles in education are those of the class teacher and support staff . . . The class teacher brings . . . specialist knowledge of the child or young person in an education context as well as expertise on the learning and teaching process.
>
> (Ibid.: 18)

Policy-articulating role specificity necessitates good knowledge exchange practices, but in practice teachers may not have contact with an AHP before classroom learning activities are initiated, nor their knowledge and skills sought in any assessment process or decision-making. Indeed, *Guidance on Partnership Working Between Allied Health Professions and Education* advises that:

> consultation time is made available in schools for staff to meet with allied health professionals and plan jointly. This may not always involve the class teacher directly, but may involve the member of staff with overall responsibility for managing support for all . . . [who] may gather the relevant information from class teachers and use this to plan jointly with the allied health professional.
>
> (Ibid.: 33)

In such a limited – or absent – relationship of knowledge and skills exchange between practitioners, the position of the teacher, then, is close to that of technician, where, in a very restricted bridging social capital relation, just enough knowledge is transferred to implement activities planned by others: a relationship which does not recognize or capitalize upon teachers' knowledge and skills, with potentially negative effects for transprofessional practice. A comment by an AHP illustrates the difficulties they experience when teachers are unconnected, or at critical times disconnected, from the knowledge exchange networks for the child:

> It is everyone's responsibility to communicate what their role is – not for others to try and work it out.
>
> (Ibid.: 19)

And a response by *Enquire: The Scottish Advice Service for Additional Support for Learning* further states (ibid: 19):

> What comes over from our helpline is that too many assumptions are made about roles.

Dysfunction and disconnect in the 'teacher as assistant'/AHP operational level relationship is exacerbated where the AHP's subject disciplinary knowledge, for example, concerning linguistics or dietetics is privileged over the teacher's knowledge of the child. AHPs employ an 'assess-intervene-reassess' paradigm not unknown in schools, but using measurements that may be unfamiliar to teachers and with access to therapies and techniques potentially beneficial to children that differ from usual classroom practice. Such intervention programmes need to be accompanied by the institution of strong bridging transprofessional relations. Instituting relations between practitioners, which legitimate knowledge exchange through adequate 'consultation time' (ibid.: 33) and allow the AHP/teacher 'to share knowledge and skills' (ibid.: 19) at all stages of an intervention (see, for example, Forbes 2008), is key for such interventions to succeed. Otherwise, where practitioner consultation and collaboration are lacking the potentially beneficial disciplinary knowledge and skills of the AHP/teacher will not be exchanged, or will be transferred perhaps less than adequately by, for example, service or school managers.

An integration policy misaligned with separate or limited joint practice produces relational disconnects where the classroom teacher may be asked to carry out activities only after a child has been referred to and assessed by an AHP, after parents and the head teacher have agreed to a school-based intervention, and after further assessments and meetings have taken place, all without the teacher's involvement in these knowledge-exchange relations. Excluded from such knowledge exchange and decision-making networks, teachers are then charged to deliver intervention. It would be unsurprising if this relationship disconnect resulted in critical omissions and gaps in the knowledge gathered, a lack of understanding or ownership of the planned intervention activities by teachers, and an inability to initiate and build the kinds of strong transprofessional social capital relations that would optimally benefit the child user of the joint service. Such a lack of shared material knowledge, and weak and inadequate transprofessional bridging and linking social capital, critically undermines the effective operation of the roles of the teacher and AHP and potentially puts in jeopardy the likelihood of getting right transprofessional trans-sectoral working for every child.

Concluding reflections, questions and suggestions

This analysis would suggest that careful scrutiny of education, health and social policy and professional governance and guidance is needed for its divergences likely to produce effects in practices that are coherent or disconnected. This examination identified tensions between policy rhetoric of partnership and/or collaboration and/or integration. The inconsistencies, incoherencies and disconnects such mixed messages produce in practice relations to the dis-benefit of service users suggest that the moment is opportune for transdisciplinary studies which closely examine the materiality of the forms of practitioner relations now operating in cross-boundary trans-sectoral working. Such studies, critically gathering the views of all practitioners involved in new practice relations and using a relational framework such as that offered by social capital theory to examine the materiality of the forms of practitioner relations, would serve to feed some important messages upstream to the children's services policy and governance community.

It is suggested that such a new conceptualization and analytic for *transprofessional relations* in policy practice and knowledge exchange is now urgently needed. As here, analysing actual integration-in-practice relations in detail might reveal how social capital is established, is deployed and breaks down – what has been termed the 'dark side' of social capital (Portes 1998). For example, where intra- (within) agency bonding capital operates in ways that are 'Balkanized' or in silos exclusive of other agency practitioners and so potentially limits the range and quality of the joint services offered to children and families. There is, of course, much more to develop in this kind of mapping and analysis of the spatiality of social capital, but it does signal some points for closer scrutiny in the interstices in which the glue of social capital is formed or not; and in so doing its application may be productive.

Heuristic use of the frame of social capital in studies to identify and analyse current relations and connections at the intersections of sub-types and key terms at each of these levels may identify where, on the basis of knowledge from transdisciplinary research, relations need to be reconceptualized and remade for the benefit of service users (and practitioners). Such a focus, albeit heuristically, on the interstices at the junctions of bonding, bridging and linking social capital in relation to practitioner networks might provoke the following questions (adapted from Forbes, 2011):

- Are practitioners' professional practice and knowledge exchange networks exclusively bonding in nature – delimited to one's own profession/discipline and excluding other practitioner groups?
- Where issues cross agency boundaries and are cross-cutting, do practitioners and sectors initiate and sustain reciprocal networks of practice and knowledge exchange that bridge to other services and include practitioners and/or leaders from other professional groups as appropriate and necessary for the benefit of the users of their joint service?

- Does children's sector agency governance and regulation institute strong linked policy arena networks that include practitioners equally with leaders and managers amongst all agencies involved in the service of children?

Concerns and dangers in merging services and integrating their operations are many. For example, the effects of the *eCare Framework* and programme (SG 2006) for service users and practitioners and the uses to which the data it holds are put must be closely scrutinized. Integration may not solve previous problems of gaps and/or overlaps in service and in doing so may indeed create new problems to do with creating a service so big and complex that it is too hard to manage. Importantly, policy, and policy technology, such as that related to eCare, must not either run too far ahead of practice or, where giving messages to a professional sector, rearticulate previous discourses at odds with the main stream and trajectories of integration policy. And where evidence demonstrates that convergence and the formation of new transprofessional social capital relations is likely to be beneficial to users then service integration and its good operation must not be blocked or fudged by defensive restrictive or protective professional regulation.

References

Baron, S., Field, J. and Schuller, T. (eds) (2000) *Social capital: critical perspectives*, Oxford: Oxford University Press.
Bourdieu, P. (1977a) *Outline of a theory of practice*, Cambridge: Cambridge University Press.
—— (1977b) 'Cultural reproduction and social reproduction', in J. Karabel and A. H. Halsey (eds) *Power and ideology in education*, Oxford: Oxford University Press.
—— (1986) 'The forms of capital', in J. G. Richardson (ed.) *Handbook of theory and research for the sociology of education*, New York: Greenwood.
—— (1993) *The field of cultural production*, Oxford: Polity Press.
Brown, K. and White, W. (2006) *Exploring the evidence base for integrated children's services*, Edinburgh: Scottish Executive.
Coleman, J. S. (1988) 'Social capital in the creation of human capital', *American Journal of Sociology* 94 (Supplement): S95–S120.
—— (1990) *Foundations of social theory*, Cambridge, MA: Bellnap Press/Harvard University Press.
Department for Children Schools and Families (DCSF) (2008a) *The Bercow Report: a review of services for children and young people (0–19) with speech, language and communication needs*, Nottingham: DCSF Publications. Online. Available at: www.dcsf.gov.uk/bercow review (accessed 17 November 2009).
—— (2008b) *Building brighter futures: next steps for the children's workforce*, London: The Stationery Office.
Department of Education (DE) (Northern Ireland) (2005) *Draft supplementary guidance to support the impact of SENDO on the code of practice on the identification and assessment of special educational needs*, Bangor: Department of Education.
Department for Education and Skills (DfES) (2004) *Every child matters: change for children*, London: DfES.
—— (2005) *Children's workforce strategy*, London: DfES.

Field, J. (2009) 'A social capital toolkit for schools? Organizational perspectives on current social capital research', in J. Allan, J. Ozga, J. Smith and G. Smith (eds) *Social capital, professionalism and diversity*, London: Routledge.

Forbes, J. (2008) 'Knowledge transformations: examining the knowledge needed in teacher and speech and language therapist co-work', *Educational Review* 60: 141–54.

—— (2011) 'Interprofessional capital in children's services transformations', *International Journal of Inclusive Education* 15(5): 573–88.

Forbes, J. and Watson, C. (eds) (2009) *Service integration in schools: research and policy discourses, practices and future prospects*, Rotterdam: Sense.

General Teaching Council for Scotland (GTCS) (2006) *Driving forward professional standards for teachers. The Standard for Full Registration*, Edinburgh: GTCS.

Grek, S., Ozga, J. and Lawn, M. (2009) *Integrated children's services in Scotland: Project KNOWandPOL Orientation 2*. Online. Available at: http://www.ces.ed.ac.uk/PDF%20Files/K%2BPPA01.pdf (accessed 9 September 2010).

Halpern, D. (2005) *Social capital*, Cambridge: Polity Press.

Hartley, D. (2009) 'Education policy and the "inter" regnum', in J. Forbes and C. Watson (eds) *Service integration in schools: research and policy discourses, practices and future prospects*, Rotterdam: Sense.

Health Professions Council (HPC) (2007) *Standards of proficiency: speech and language therapists*. Online. Available at: http://www.hpc-uk.org/assets/documents/10000529Standards_of_Proficiency_SLTs.pdf (accessed 9 September 2010).

Her Majesty's Inspectorate of Education (HMIE) (2002) *Count us in – achieving inclusion in Scottish schools*, Edinburgh: The Stationery Office.

—— (2005) *A common approach to inspecting services for children and young people*, Edinburgh: Scottish Executive.

—— (2007) *Report on the implementation of the Education (Additional Support for Learning) (Scotland) Act 2004*. Online. Available at: http://www.hmie.gov.uk/documents/publication/aslr.pdf (accessed 7 September 2010).

—— (2009) *Improving Scottish education: a report by HMIE on inspection and review 2005–2008*, Livingston: HMIE.

Narayan, D. (1999) *Bonds and bridges: social capital and poverty*, Washington, DC: World Bank.

Office of the First Minister and Deputy First Minister (OFMDFM) (2006) *Our children and young people: our pledge. A ten year strategy for children and young people in Northern Ireland, 2006–2016*, Belfast: OFMDFM.

Organization for Economic Co-operation and Development (OECD) (2000) *The wealth of nations: the role of human and social capital*, Paris: OECD.

Percy-Smith, J. (2005) *What works in strategic partnerships for children?* Barkingside: Barnardo's.

Portes, A. (1998) 'Social capital: its origins and applications in modern sociology', *Annual Review of Sociology* 24: 1–24.

Putnam, R. D. (1993) *Making democracy work: civic traditions in modern Italy*, Princeton, NJ: Princeton University Press.

—— (1995) 'Tuning in, tuning out: the strange disappearance of social capital in America', *Political Science and Politics* 28: 1–20.

—— (2000) *Bowling alone: the collapse and revival of American community*, New York: Simon and Schuster.

Scottish Executive (SE) (2000) *Making a difference: effective implementation of cross-cutting policy*, Edinburgh, Policy Review Unit: Scottish Executive.

—— (2001) *For Scotland's children: better integrated children's services*, Edinburgh: Scottish Executive.

—— (2005) *Getting it right for every child: proposals for action*, Edinburgh: Scottish Executive.

—— (2006a) *A guide to evaluating services for children and young people using quality indicators*, Edinburgh: Scottish Executive.

—— (2006b) *The code of practice for the joint inspection of services to protect children and young people*, Edinburgh: Scottish Executive. Online. Available at: http://www.scotland.gov/Resource/Doc/117372/0028869.pdf (accessed 10 March 2008).

Scottish Executive Education Department (SEED) (2006) *Improving outcomes for children and young people: the role of schools in delivering integrated children's services*, Edinburgh: Scottish Executive Education Department.

Scottish Government (SG) (2006) *Promotional leaflet for launch of eCare Framework 1.0*, Edinburgh: Scottish Government. Online. Available at: http://www.scotland.gov.uk/Publications/2006/05/11150808/1 (accessed 9 September 2010).

—— (2008) *Getting it Right For Every Child (GiRFEC) overview*. Online. Available at: http://www.scotland.gov.uk/Topics/People/Young-People/childrenservices/girfec/programme-overview (accessed 17 November 2009).

—— (2010) *Guidance on partnership working between allied health professions and education*, Edinburgh: Scottish Government.

Scottish Office (SO) (1998) *New community schools: the prospectus*. Online. Available at: http://www.scotland.gov.uk/library/documents-w3/ncsp-00.htm (accessed 21 June 2008).

Scottish Parliament (SP) (2006) *Joint inspection of services for children and inspection of social work services (Scotland) Act*, Edinburgh: Scottish Parliament.

Teacher Development Agency (TDA) (2007) *Professional standards for teachers. Why sit still in your career?* Online. Available at: http://www.tda.gov.uk/upload/resources/pdf/t/tda 0313%20%20professional%20standards%20for%20teachers.pdf (accessed 9 September 2010).

UK Government Performance and Innovation Unit (2002) *Social capital: a discussion paper*, London: Performance and Innovation Unit.

UK Parliament (2004) *Children Act (England) (2004)*, London: The Stationery Office.

United States 107th Congress (2002) *An act to close the achievement gap with accountability, flexibility and choice, so that no child is left behind. This title may be cited as the 'No child left behind act of 2001' Public Law 107–10*, Washington: US Congress. Online. Available at: http://www2.ed.gov/policy/elsec/leg/esea02/107-110.pdf (accessed 7 August 2010).

Chapter 5

For whom the bell tolls

Education, care and the possibility of
professional practice in uncertain times

Ian Stronach and John Clarke

> The end had come but it was not yet in sight.
> (Galbraith [2009] *The Great Crash 1929*: 86)

Introduction

Forget the Twin Towers. Recall, instead, the collapse of Communism in 1989 – that
was an historic event, taking down with it the epistemological tower of 'scientific
socialism' (Engels 2008); 150 years of a certain kind of utopian nightmare came to
an end, along with its half-forgotten dreams. Recall, also, the 'Great Recession' of
2008 when down came the even older parallel tower of 'scientific capitalism'.[1]
Together these two collapses mark out the territory of the 21st century – which is
only now beginning.

> The credit crunch was not just a financial collapse, but the collapse of an ideology
> – that the wider and deeper markets became the greater the public good.
> (Graham 2009)

Between them, an old and recurrent positivism also crumbles. The science of the
social is once again (but surely not for ever) made implausible by a world that keeps
on demonstrating its unpredictability, the failure of its quantitative reduction to the
certainties of rules, patterns and paradigms, the absence of our control over its
'outputs'.[2] When the markets crashed, certain forms of thinking tumbled with them
in ways that we need to mark, for it is always true that collective amnesia attends such
historic events and their consequences. Indeed, its 'green shoots' are already hard at
work. The implications of these changes are radical for all spheres of education and
social care, since a kind of methodological reductionism and instrumentality is
common to many manifestations of contemporary professional policy, discourse and
practice. Indeed there are signs that a greater instrumentalism will result – in line with
the sort of thinking Festinger, Rieken and Schachter (1956) identified in *When
prophecy fails*, the failure of the system of belief to correspond with reality *tightens*
belief in its inevitability.

But we need to start at the beginning, which already lies well behind us. What was
the scale and import of the economic collapse? What can be learned from capitalist

comment on recent events? Soros claims nothing less than 'the end of an era' (2008: 83): 'we are facing a deep and long recession, possibly amounting to a depression' (ibid.: 163). We have apparently entered a 'new stage in human history' (Gamble 2009: 166). Adair Turner, Chairman of the Financial Services Authority (FSA), the UK financial regulatory body, pronounces the 'biggest crisis in the history of market capitalism' (quoted in Parker 2009: n.p.); 'casino capitalism' is condemned (Gamble 2009: 54).

Gordon Brown, then Chancellor of the Exchequer, boasted that 'a new world order' had been created, 'a new golden age for the City of London' (Brown 2007). What is important to register is that right up to the Crash, ruling politicians in the UK and the US were claiming that *Boom and Bust* had gone for good, replaced by 'an almost messianic faith in markets' (Lee 2009: 109). Alongside such certainty was a parallel and related conviction that quantitative ingenuity had solved the problem of 'risk' in the markets. The Gaussian copula and innovative statistics from a Lehman group, headed by David Li (Jones 2009), enabled risks to be managed globally, and guaranteed by both banks and regulators. The *quant*, 'a brand of industrial scientist who applies his mathematical models of uncertainty to financial (or socio-economic) data and complex financial instruments' (Taleb 2008: 19), was now the guarantor of risk-free investment.

'Scientific capitalism' thus guaranteed that the real economy had at last been understood as an 'efficient' and largely self-regulating market, wherein risk was assessed, bundled and sold. As Boltanski and Chiapello (2007: 27) pointed out well before the Crash, a capitalism without ideological competition 'displays a fragility that emerges precisely when real competitors have disappeared'. Such a capitalism '*needs* its enemies' (ibid.: 27, original emphasis). Bereft of such a corrective, the impersonalization of risk and its judgement licensed a new irresponsibility where no one knew whose risks had been bought or even – usually – how these risks had been assessed. It is significant for our overall thesis to note that such confidence in the financial-statistical construction of economic knowledge overlapped into other disciplines and discourses, where a shared 'Platonicity' (Taleb 2008: 17) and faith in normative statistical manipulation also based on the bell-shaped curve grew in popularity in the 1980s and 1990s. People were persuaded that what had come about was a 'science' of 'financial engineering' (Taleb 2007: 115). Similarly, in a metonymic extension of that faith, discourses such as education, health, medicine and their associated methodologies became populated by all sorts of economistic metaphors and assumptions – league tables, 'added-value', 'delivery', 'output', 'knowledge economy', 'measurement science' and so on (Hargreaves 1996; Soros 2008; Okagaki, Albio and Buckley 2009; Tett 2009). More materially, 'markets' or quasi-markets were created in the public sector in order to motivate and measure all sorts of professional performance. In Marxist terms such a colonization reflects the under-consumptionist thesis (Baran and Sweezy 1968), in a creeping commodification of the 'social'. As such, it was a kind of universal 'subordination to the global axiomatic of capital' (Patton 2008: 188).[3] But there was a problem with this 'knowledge economy': 'elaborate mathematical models . . . proved to be false gods' (Ferguson 2009: 14).

Such a colonization of the 'social' and the 'educational' by the 'economic' is not just political and moral in nature. It extends to the philosophically important root metaphors through which society understands itself – as in the proliferation of 'cultural capitals' and 'social capitals' in academic discourses over the last few years.[4] The market constructed a 'knowledge economy' in its own image, in a kind of commodification of epistemology and philosophy. The metaphor of the market metamorphosed into the literal. Then the market crashed, and with it the warrant for that 'scientific capitalism', but not – so far – its many simulacra in the 'managed professions' and their worlds of markets and outputs, audit and accountability. The mirror was broken, but its reflections were undisturbed. Hence, what followed was a *redoubled cargo cult* of capitalist illusion.[5]

But the world is at least predictably unpredictable. The 'Great Recession' showed once more that crisis rather than increment still defines capitalism. Once again, there was 'a generalized global crisis' (McNally 2008). The parallels with the 1929 Crash were clear, and indeed its spectre had already been raised by the dot.com bubble crash (Boyle 2000; Temin and Voth 2003).[6] There had been the same debt-fuelled speculation, the same gamble that the markets could only go on rising, the same faith in the 'science' of the trusts, and the 'magic of leverage' (Galbraith 2009: 59). Indeed, there was in the 1920s a similarly powerful opposition to regulation from the 'liquidationists' who opposed it as 'unscientific' intervention in the natural workings of the market (Parker 2008: 271–81). Coolidge, like Gordon Brown and others in 2007, stood on the cliff-edge of a Crash and saw nothing but growing prosperity: 'the highest record of years of prosperity' (Galbraith 2009: 6). Yet the banks went bang, Coolidge departed, and Brown resumed his tragicomic descent from Old Labour to New Labour to No Labour. Even the aftermath of 1929 had its parallels with 2008–9. Galbraith noted wryly of that earlier period: 'Such was the fate of the bankers. For the next decade they were fair game for Congressional committees, courts, the press, and the comedians' (ibid.: 136). Then as now.

He also noted that at least the 'gargantuan insanity' of the 1920s boom had led to an 'immunizing memory' (ibid.: 29, 89) although of course that immunity did not last through to the 21st century, when the same 'irrational exuberance' (Temin and Voth 2003: 2; Ferguson 2009: 122) surfaced again, this time often ludicrously attributed to some hard-wired neurological inevitability in man's make-up. 'Greed' became 'Nature' in the cult of the hippocampus. Overall, as Ferguson noted, 'plenty mathematics, but not enough history' (Ferguson 2009: 330); as a result of which 'markets have short memories' (ibid.: 333). Skidelsky (2009: n.p.) reached the same conclusion: 'Students of economics should be taught more history and less maths.' Suddenly, memories are temporarily restored, and the financial press recalls that history does repeat itself, even if inexactly: 'Roughly speaking, the banking world makes the same mistake every 15 or 20 years' (Henry Hoare, quoted in Murphy and Jenkins 2009: n.p.). As to how short these memories are, it is instructive that Saigol (2009: n.p.), writing in the *Financial Times*, and commenting on the stock market 'recovery' in September 2009, should begin an article with the words: 'It was almost as if the past year had never happened.'[7] Amnesia, after all, has always been an instrument of policy.

As for the new sciences of human behaviour and risk management, they too have had their recurrences. Indeed, each age seems to draw on a leading scientific innovation in order to reinvent understanding of the 'social' in that image. From Boyle's Law to the Double Helix and then on to current evolutionary biology, a scientific discovery is hailed as a new metaphor of the social, a new determinism, and latest candidate for a reductionist 'explanation'. This has a long history. In the introduction to his translation of Jean-Jacques Rousseau's *Social Contract*, Cranston (1968) notes that Francis Bacon had previously sought to bring 'science' to the absolutism of James I, just as Rousseau himself sought a thoroughly Enlightened 'universal science of the wise' (Rousseau 1984: 160).[8] Malthus had a similar ambition in relation to the interests of the wealthy of his day 'by shaping into a pseudo-scientific form the secret desires of the wealth-possessing classes' (Kropotkin 1998: 78). Colebrook has entertainingly mocked such a recurrent 'bourgeois thermodynamics' (Colebrook 2008).[9] So too, much earlier, did Swift in *Gulliver's Travels*, where the Brobdingnagian king is satirically mocked for 'not having hitherto reduced *politicks* into a *science*, as the more acute wits of Europe have done' (Swift 2007: 143).

But it was not just the rich and the powerful who sought the certainties of a science for their cause. A recursive scientism certainly invested socialism, especially 'scientific socialism' from the 1830s onwards, and is still highly visible in Mandel's relatively recent introduction to Volume 1 of Marx's *Capital* (1990), but the nature of that shared epistemological fantasy will not be explored here. Ironically, of course, just as 'scientific capitalism' went out with a bang, leaving its simulacra behind, so too did socialism come back with an equal and opposite force, in the nationalization and 'rescue' of banks, insurance companies and currencies. This was not however the return of 'scientific socialism' so much as socialism as emergency medicine. Hospital or hearse? We still have to wait and see. Suddenly, Marx – that 19th-century Frankenstein – was resurrected by the very market fundamentalism that had earlier claimed to have buried him. His ghost, in *Capital*, berates 'talk of eliminating present burdens by means of government debts which put them on the shoulders of future generations' (Marx 1990: 1084). Ring any bells? It certainly does for Bank of England Governor, Mervyn King (2009: 2) who said in a speech to Scottish business organizations, 'We shall all be paying for the impact of this crisis on the public finances for a generation.'

A final point to sum up the crisis of certainty, before we return to the central themes of uncertainty, unruliness and disruption which attend our current efforts. The economic Crash destroys certain ways of understanding the economic. No one saw it coming.[10] 'Economics' was once again discredited. Even guilty politicians, in power at the time, have abandoned the 'mathematization of economics' while remaining interestingly faithful to the need to measure everything to see if it's working.[11] But the economistic discourses, with their market assumptions and metaphors, have not crashed and possibly never will. The discourses and practices of the public sector, variously invaded, bullied and made accountable to such mechanisms and assumptions, continue to mimic the erstwhile 'efficiencies' of the market. Bust or not. What we now encounter, therefore, is a kind of new cargo cult, as a state culture continues and even intensifies worship of a discredited economic model – an irrationality well understood since Festinger *et al.*'s (1956) *When Prophecy Fails*. The Devil who had no shadow now has a shadow and no body.

So what went so wrong that made a 19th century Marx so right? Thus far, contemporary critique of 'scientific capitalism' has centred on the statistical manipulation of risk, as authors such as Anderson (2007), Soros (2008), Ferguson (2009) and Holtham (2009) have indicated. The best-known of these arguments addresses the problem of the 'outlier' or the 'black swan', pointing out that Crashes (like other cataclysmic historical events) may be discountable in terms of a normative statistics, but they nevertheless happen fairly regularly, as Marx pointed out in relation to the 19th century's global economy:

> All ideas of a common, all-embracing and far-sighted control over the production of raw materials – a control that is incompatible, by and large, with the laws of capitalist production, and hence remains forever a pious wish, or is at most confined to exceptional steps in moments of great and present danger and perplexity – all such ideas give way to the belief that supply and demand will mutually regulate each other.
>
> (Marx 1991: 215)[12]

So it was not that the 'unthinkable' hadn't been thought before. Soros has concluded that the problem of certainty rests on the recurring fantasy of a science of the social: 'Anthropologists and most sociologists do not even try to imitate the natural sciences. But they are less influential than those who try' (Soros 2008: 9).

In a similar vein Taleb attacks 'scientism', particularly as it is applied within economics: 'The world is far too complicated for their discipline' (Taleb 2008: 155). Several authors have also pointed out that the element of luck and chance in markets and in social life more generally is neglected, a point now picked up in the financial press: 'Top performers will tend to have been lucky in the past, and luck rarely lasts' (Harford 2009). Game theory is an inadequate response to such complexity: 'all theories built around the ludic fallacy ignore a layer of uncertainty' (Taleb 2008: 287). Part of the problem of uncertainty lies in the nature of the unfolding of historical events. What happened ignores everything that failed to happen. Thus events readily become the 'effects' of the things that occur before them, whose correlation becomes evidence of cause. Taleb calls this 'survivorship bias' (Taleb 2007: 149). He offers a remedy – 'take a look at the cemetery' (Taleb 2008: 105). Soros' (2008) conclusion is that evolutionary biology comes closer than physics as an instructive intellectual role model. His answer to indeterminacy is to shift scientific metaphor – drawing on evolutionary biology rather than more static Newtonian models. This seems to us, however, to remain a kind of scientific tourism. A new and more exotically dynamic location, perhaps, but the same old ontological assumption. The need to include 'chance' and 'event' in accounts of the social is not new – Hayek and Nancy have written about it from Right and Left (Stronach 2008, 2010), and Keynes gives a very relevant account of how 'animal spirits' can upset the precarious 'convention' (2009: 130–1) of stable and predictable markets: 'A conventional valuation which is established as the outcome of the mass psychology of a large number of ignorant individuals is liable to change violently . . .' (ibid.: 124). It is important to remind ourselves that such changes are always subject to a recurrent and insistent amnesia.

To sum up: we did our sums wrong; we did the wrong sums. But it goes much further than that. As Keynes pointed out, the snag with history is that 'the sample size is effectively one' (cited in Ferguson 2009: 344). In addition, true experiments are seldom possible or replicable. The problem is not just that the history of the world is the wrong shape and course for statistical measurement and prediction, so much as historical events, like 'May 1968' – to give Deleuze's example – always *break* with a certain causality: 'Yet the event is itself a splitting off from, or a breaking with, causality' (Deleuze 2007: 233).

Indeed, Nancy argues similarly that the nature of 'event' as 'surprise' is inherent in the movements of the social and the historical (Nancy 1993). In the broadest terms we might contrast philosophies of the Same (universal, transcendent) with philosophies of Difference (singular, imbued with the Nietzschean Eternal Return), in the manner of Deleuze in *Difference and Repetition* (1994).

The twin towers of 'scientific socialism' and 'scientific capitalism' were always interested in resurrecting forms of positivism with which to bolster their fantasies of order, progress and predictability. The lessons of 1929, 1968 and 2008 are both well known and well forgotten. The present situation is clear, the future is not. On the one hand, the people through the agency of government rescue capitalism in 2008. The government through the agency of capital then makes the *people* repay that loan. *The debtor demands repayment.*[13] There can be no more uncertain a premise for the future than that.

What now? We are left with educational and social practices and discourses that hark back to assumptions of economic reality which proved illusory. Our 'knowledge economy' is largely founded on a cargo cult. Yet the twin towers of 'scientific socialism' and 'scientific capitalism' are always interested in resurrecting forms of positivism with which to bolster fantasies of order, progress and predictability. So we can probably assume that the 'Great Recession' will reproduce itself after a period of functional amnesia. Indeed, pro-capitalist newspapers like the *Financial Times* readily make such a prediction (for example, Authers 2010a, 2010b). As Festinger *et al.* (1956) long ago pointed out in relation to prophecy and prediction, evidence of refutation can strengthen belief. Or is it just possible that the cult of 'economy' worship that has been hegemonic for so long has lost its powers of both persuasion and amnesia?

This has been a preliminary attempt to sketch out the political and contemporary dilemma for 'knowledge production', or 'knowledge labour' as we might want to call it, in relation to qualitative inquiry in the 21st century.[14] It underpins, of course, any possibility of professional practice in a new context. It is a move away from a 'prefigurable' history (Negri 2008: 38). Our goal: to put Uncertainty back on her throne, perhaps recalling Proudhon: 'Anarchy is order, government is civil war' (quoted in Kinna 2005: 5). Such novel appropriations of concepts more conventionally treated separately and in polar terms are also attempts for some at least to 'snatch Marxism back from its scientific status', in terms similar to Negri's ambition (Negri 2008: 130). What for? To work for 'the invention of a new form of freedom' (ibid: 158).

Notes

1 So-called; see, for example, Lemer (2009).
2 There is also a perennial confusion of 'outputs' with 'outcomes', the former marking something of the industrialization of life, learning and affect.
3 As Lather (2009: 2) notes, some have seen in this a 'vast neoliberal conspiracy'. But there are as many elements of cock-up as conspiracy. And both terms fail to catch both the functional nature of the cargo cult (Worsley 1970) that was engendered and the diminished economic role of the 'hollowed-out' state – a circumstance which encouraged politicians to move the levers they could still reach – 'education, education, education', as UK premier Tony Blair famously said in setting out his political agenda.
4 Steve Baron (2009) noted 17 different 'capitals' deployed in social science and education.
5 Cargo cults in the South Sea Islands were a ritualized nostalgia for departed prosperity, mainly US bases in WWII (Worsley 1970). They enacted in dance, for example, the flight of bombers and hence recalled the ephemeral wealth of having US bases in their midst (Harris 1989). The related game of Trobriand cricket, however, is perhaps the most well-known exemplar of this kind of ritual mimicry.
6 Boyle's article could not have been more explicit: 'Are we facing another Wall Street Crash?'(Boyle 2000). It could be argued that Alan Greenspan (Chairman US Federal Reserve 1987–2006) successfully postponed an affirmative answer to that question, but by 2008 it was becoming inevitable.
7 To be fair to the *Financial Times*, their editorial take is firmly pessimistic, as they sense that the VW dilemma regarding the shape of the recession is driving towards the W: 'Where have all the green shoots gone?' (Anon. 2009: n.p.).
8 It should be acknowledged that the word 'science' carried a different weight at that time and could be used by undetermined and undetermining philosophers like Hume in the sense of a more general 'knowledge' (Hume 2004).
9 Such 'thermodynamic' argumentation reduces difference to a 'quantification of "intensities" in an economy of more or less' (Colebrook 2008: 130).
10 Not quite true, of course. In any distribution of opinion, there will always be some 'outlier' predictions that turn out to be 'black swans'. Marxists could make such a claim, of course, if they hadn't spent so much of the last 150 years with that other animal harbinger, 'crying wolf'. As Wheen points out, Marx hurried to finish the *Grundrisse* before the onset of the 'deluge' (Wheen 1999: 243). There were also pro-market dissidents, like Roubini in the US and Cable in the UK (Brockes 2009; Cable 2009).
11 Charles Clarke, former Labour minister, speaking on BBC Radio 4's 'Start the week' programme, 11 January 2011.
12 Marx returned to mark the tragedy of the 2008 Crash, but also suitably returned again as farce. A hoax Marx passage from *Capital* was circulated on Wall Street (Rainey 2009). And a musical in China. And a manga [comic], *Capital*, in Japan.
13 Many have noted the irony of capitalism for the profits, and socialism for the losses – actually on both Left and Right in the US and the UK. Hutton (2009) estimates future UK taxpayer-incurred debt as a result of the 'rescue' to be between £50 and £100 billion. In a lighter pre-Christmas mood, the *Financial Times* satirized the situation via the parable of 'Consumerella'. The fable ends thus: 'It was only in January that Consumerella's credit card statement arrived and she discovered that Santa Claus had paid for the gifts by taking out a loan in her name. They all lived miserably ever after. The End.' (Harford 2008: n.p.).
14 A metaphorical (and political) shift from 'capital' to 'labour' would meet with the approval of Marx, but also with the beliefs of Adam Smith: 'Labour, therefore, it appears evidently, is the only universal, as well as the only accurate measure of value' (Smith 2008: 42).

References

Anderson, C. (2007) *The long tail. How endless choice is creating unlimited demand*, London: Random House.

Anon. (2009) 'Where have all the green shoots gone?', *Financial Times*, 23 October. Online. Available at: http://www.ft.com/cms/s/0/c3c8274a-c002-11de-aed2-00144feab49a. html#axzz1HKwfGzGx (accessed 23 March 2011).

Authers, J. (2010a) 'Chance to make system safer may have been lost', *Financial Times*, 18 September. Online. Available at: http://www.ft.com/cms/s/0/5db36668-c2a4-11df-956e-00144feab49a.html (accessed 18 March 2011).

—— (2010b) 'Finreg heralds a Great Escape for bankers', *Financial Times*, 16 July. Online. Available at: http://www.ft.com/cms/s/0/2a1c6958-9112-11df-b297-00144feab49a. html#axzz1GxdO0RgA (accessed 18 March 2011).

Baran, P. and Sweezy, P. (1968) *Monopoly capital*, New York: Review Press.

Baron, S. (2009) 'Social theory and the spawning of capitals', paper presented at ESRC seminar series: Confluences of identity, knowledge and practice: building interprofessional social capital, University of Aberdeen, May 2009.

Boltanski, L. and Chiapello, E. (2007) *The new spirit of capitalism*, London: Verso.

Boyle, D. (2000) 'Are we facing another Wall Street Crash?', *Ecologist* 1: 11. Online. Available at: www.neweconomics.org/gen/m6_i63_news.aspx (accessed 15 July 2009).

Brockes, E. (2009) 'He told us so', *Guardian*, 24 January. Online. Available at: http:// www.guardian.co.uk/business/2009/jan/24/nouriel-roubini-credit-crunch (accessed 26 march 2011).

Brown, G. (2007) Speech by the Chancellor of the Exchequer, the Rt Hon. Gordon Brown MP, Mansion House, 20 June 2007. Online. Available at: http://webarchive.national archives.gov.uk/+/http://www.hm-treasury.gov.uk/newsroom_and_speeches/press /2007/press_68_07.cfm (accessed 18 March 2011).

Cable, V. (2009) *The storm – world crisis and what it means*, London: Atlantic.

Colebrook, C. (2008) 'Bourgeois thermodynamics', in I. Buchanan and N. Thorborn (eds) *Deleuze and politics*, Edinburgh: Edinburgh University Press.

Cranston, M. (1968) 'Introduction', in J.-J. Rousseau *The social contract*, London: Penguin.

Deleuze, G. (1994) *Difference and repetition*, London: Athlone Press.

—— (2007) *Two regimes of madness. Texts and interviews 1975–95*, Paris: Semiotext(e).

Engels, F. (2008 [1907]) *Landmarks of scientific socialism*, New York: Cosimo.

Ferguson, N. (2009) *The ascent of money. A financial history of the world*, London: Penguin.

Festinger, L., Rieken, H. and Schachter, S. (1956) *When prophecy fails. A social and psychological study of a group that predicted the destruction of the world*, London: Harper and Row.

Galbraith, K. (2009 [1954]) *The Great Crash 1929*, London: Penguin.

Gamble, A. (2009) *The spectre at the feast. Capitalist crisis and the politics of recession*, London: Palgrave Macmillan.

Graham, A. (2009) Comment on 'Lehman's – one year on: have we learned the lessons?' *Guardian* Roundtable, 15 September. Online. Available at: http://www.guardian.co.uk/ commentisfree/2009/sep/14/lehmans-one-year-after (accessed 23 March 2011).

Harford, T. (2008) 'Is the credit crunch suitable for children?', *Financial Times*, 12 December. Online. Available at: http://www.ft.com/cms/s/2/a2321930-c65f-11dd-a741-000077 b07658.html#axzz1HKwfGzGx (accessed 22 March 2011).

—— (2009) 'To profit, plump for an also-ran at the helm', *Financial Times*, 25 April. Online. Available at: http://www.ft.com/cms/s/2/3ec5a0bc-2d73-11de-9eba-00144feabdc0. html#axzz1HKwfGzGx (accessed 13 January 2011).

Hargreaves, D. (1996) 'Teaching as a research-based profession', annual lecture Teacher Training Agency, London. Online. Available at: http://www.bera.ac.uk/files/resources files/educationalresearch/hargreaves_1996.pdf (accessed 23 March 2011).

Harris, M. (1989) *Cows, pigs, wars, and witches. The riddles of culture*, New York: Vintage.

Holtham, G. (2009) *Global dimension of the financial crisis*, London: Institute for Public Policy Research. Online. Available at: http://www.ippr.org.uk/members/download.asp? f=%2Fecomm%2Ffiles%2Fglobal%5Fdimensions%5Ffinancial%5Fcrisis%2Epdf (accessed 24 March 2011).

Hume, D. (2004) *An enquiry concerning human understanding*, New York: Dover Publications.

Hutton, W. (2009) 'High stakes, low finance', The *Guardian*, 2 May. Online. Available at: http://www.guardian.co.uk/books/2009/may/02/big-bang-will-hutton (accessed 24 March 2011).

Jones. S. (2009) 'The formula that felled Wall St', *Financial Times*, 24 April. Online. Available at: http://www.ft.com/cms/s/2/912d85e8-2d75-11de-9eba-00144feabdc0.html#axzz 1HKwfGzGx (accessed 24 March 2011).

Keynes, J. (2009) *The general theory of employment, interest and money*, New York: Classic Books America.

King, M. (2009) Speech by Mervyn King, Governor of the Bank of England to Scottish business organisations, Edinburgh, 20 October 2009. Online. Available at: http://www. bankofengland.co.uk/publications/speeches/2009/speech406.pdf (accessed 27 February 2011).

Kinna, R. (2005) *Anarchism. A beginner's guide*, Oxford: Oneworld.

Kropotkin, N. (1998 [1898]) *Fields, factories and workshops tomorrow*, London: Freedom House.

Lather, P. (2009) 'Scientism and scientificity in the rage for accountability', in R. St Clair (ed.) *Education science. Critical perspectives*, Rotterdam: Sense.

Lee, S. (2009) *Boom and bust. The problems and legacy of Gordon Brown*, Oxford: Oneworld.

Lemer, J. (2009) 'The big stories', *Financial Times*, 25 April. Online. Available at: http:// www.ft.com/cms/s/0/d612e96e-3130-11de-8196-00144feabdc0.html#axzz1HKwf GzGx (accessed 22 March 2011).

McNally, D. (2008) 'From financial crisis to world slump: accumulation, financialization, and the global slowdown'. Online. Available at: http://marx and the financialcrisisof2008.blog spot.com/2008/12/david-mcnally-from-financial-crisis-to.html (accessed 15 September 2009).

Marx, K. (1990 [1867]) *Capital: a critique of political economy. Volume 1*, London: Penguin/New Left Review.

—— (1991 [1894]) *Capital. A critique of political economy. Volume 3*, London: Penguin/New Left Review.

Murphy, M. and Jenkins, P. (2009) 'Experienced banker exudes sang-froid', *Financial Times*, 2 October. Online. Available at: http://www.ft.com/cms/s/0/11ae5d6a-af7a-11de-ba1c-00144feabdc0.html#axzz1HKwfGzGx (accessed 22 March 2011).

Nancy, J.-L. (1993) *The experience of freedom*, Stanford: Stanford University Press.

Negri, A. (2008) *Reflections on 'Empire'*, London: Polity Press.

Okagaki, L., Albio, E. and Buckley, J. (2009) 'Institute of Education Sciences – putting science back into education research', in R. St Clair (ed.) *Education science. Critical perspectives*, Rotterdam: Sense.

Parker, G. (2009) 'City "failing to learn lessons of crisis"', *Financial Times*, 23 June. Online. Available at:<http://www.ft.com/cms/s/0/13ce71c6-5fdd-11de-a09b-00144feabdc0, s01=1.html#axzz1HKwfGzGx (accessed 13 January 2011).

Parker, S. (2008) *The Great Crash. How the stock market crash of 1929 plunged the world into depression*, London: Little Brown/Piatkus.

Patton, P. (2008) 'Becoming-democratic', in I. Buchanan and N. Thorborn (eds) *Deleuze and Politics*, Edinburgh: Edinburgh University Press.

Rainey, M. (2009) 'Wall Street's Marxist moment'. Online. Available at: http://www.bloggingstocks.com/2009/01/26/wall-streets-marxist-moment/ (accessed (15 September 2009).

Rousseau, J.-J. (1984) *A discourse on inequality*, London: Penguin.

Saigol, L. (2009) 'Raised spirits', *Financial Times*, 11 September. Online. Available at: http://www.ft.com/cms/s/0/9faf2514-9f0c-11de-8013-00144feabdc0.html#axzz1HKwfGzGx (accessed 11 March 2011).

Skidelsky, R. (2009) Comment on 'Lehman's – one year on: have we learned the lessons?', The *Guardian* Roundtable, 15 September. Online. Available at: http://www.guardian.co.uk/commentisfree/2009/sep/14/lehmans-one-year-after (accessed 23 March 2011).

Smith, A. (2008 [1776]) *An enquiry into the nature and causes of the wealth of nations. A selected edition*, in K. Sutherland (ed.), Oxford: Oxford University Press.

Soros, G. (2008) *The Crash of 2008*, New York: Public Affairs.

Stronach, I. (2008) 'Rethinking words, concepts, stories and theories', address to the International Congress of Qualitative Inquiry, University of Illinois (Urbana-Champaign), May 2008.

—— (2010) *Globalizing education, educating the local: how method made us mad*, London: Routledge.

Swift, J. (2007 [1726]) *Gulliver's travels: and Alexander Pope's Verses on Gulliver's travels*, London: Vintage.

Taleb, N. (2007) *Fooled by randomness. The hidden role of chance in life and the markets*, 2nd Edition, London: Penguin.

—— (2008) *The black swan: the impact of the highly improbable*, London: Penguin.

Temin, P. and Voth, H.-J. (2003) 'Riding the South Sea Bubble', Masachussetts Institute of Technology, Dept of Economics. Online. Available at: http://ssrn.com/abstract=485482) (accessed 15 July 2009).

Tett, G. (2009) *Fool's gold. How unrestrained greed corrupted a dream, shattered global markets and unleashed a catastrophe*, London: Little Brown.

Wheen, F. (1999) *Karl Marx*, London: Fourth Estate.

Worsley, P. (1970 [1957]) *The trumpet shall sound: a study of cargo cults in Melanesia*, London: Paladin.

Part III

Preparing practitioners and leaders for inter/professional practice

Identities, connections, knowledges

Chapter 6

Social capital connections

Troublesome knowledge and early career practitioners

James McGonigal and Julie McAdam

Introduction

If effective inter/professional working is to develop between those who work with children and young people in various educational and care contexts, then some sort of shared 'theory' is needed. Theory here is taken to mean a rationale that is assented to by the different professionals involved in such working together, and a felt awareness of the attitudes, values and constraints that operate within their different contexts. Social capital theory offers one perspective but is a concept which is under-researched (if often cited) in professional contexts. In these overlapping and sensitive areas of professional life, social capital theory might provide at least a framework for thinking about the social issues of poverty and alienation that often bring teachers and social workers (for example) together.

Yet because social capital operates as a heuristic device at a certain level of generality (more effectively deployed at the macro level of policy or the meso level of reflection, rather than at the micro level of practice) it may need an additional theoretical frame to maximize its potential to explore the hard actualities of professional decision-making. Here we offer such a theory, one that is currently used to think about conceptual difficulties and, increasingly, professional learning across a range of academic disciplines. The notions of 'troublesome knowledge' and 'threshold concepts' can perhaps offer a shared language in which the next generation of teachers and social workers can begin to understand each others' aims and intentions.

The role of the educators and mentors of these new 'inter/professionals', in both higher education and in practice situations, would then become akin to that of translators, ensuring that professional signs (events, disagreements, comments, intuitions) are accurately heard and understood, and appropriately responded to. Before such effective and genuine engagement can begin to take place across the 'caring disciplines', it is the tutors themselves who need to gain fluency not only in the discourses that they may already share but also in the various professional dialects that they do not yet fully comprehend. They are best placed to shape the educative experiences that beginning teachers or social workers undergo, and also the language that these early-stage professionals begin to understand and use as they enter more confidently into professional and inter/professional life.

Social capital in professional contexts

Professional induction cannot be seen simply as a passive process of transmission and reception of craft, knowledge and skills. It also involves values and attitudes and an openness to reflection on the process of one's own learning. In education (the discipline that the current authors are most familiar with on a daily working basis), becoming professional is an interactive process in which there often occurs a challenging dialogue between the beginning teacher's confidence in the discourse and content of a subject specialism or social/vocational aspiration ('I want to be a really good teacher of physics'; 'I want to help young children learn to read') and the sometimes contradictory voices of colleagues, fellow students, mentors and also children within the context of classroom experience. The notion of threshold concepts in teaching and learning can provide insights into this dialogic process of adjustment between intention and actual effect, and also into ways in which institutions involved in the education of teachers or social workers might handle the problems encountered in becoming a professional.

This chapter builds on an earlier research project that attempted to identify social capital, threshold concepts and troublesome knowledge in teacher education, to consider how these relate to subject knowledge, and to explore whether such concepts, once identified, might be effectively used to reshape the content or process of the Postgraduate Certificate in Education (PGCE) courses and the year-long school-based probationer training that follows (Cove, McAdam and McGonigal 2008a). Exploring the place of values, dispositions and relationships within early professional work contexts, the project led us towards a clarification of the types of social capital created by the processes and practice of teacher education, conceived as an interactive continuum between individual and community aspirations and needs. The ideas of social capital already demanded critique across a range of social and caring professions and we were interested in the various ways in which student teachers seek and find guidance or other sorts of social support, or indeed come to sustain each other in their new professional role.

Social capital theory with its focus on networks, norms, trust and reciprocity offers a new way of thinking about the relational dimensions of learning to teach, and about how teachers during their early professional life begin to relate to a widening range of colleagues, and also to make more effective links to the local communities whose children they serve. This is particularly important in the current policy context of social inclusion and inter/professional working and the professional mentoring of new teachers in Scottish schools through the probation experience monitored by the General Teaching Council for Scotland (GTCS); and is of concern beyond the period of professional probation for individuals' continuing professional formation. In all of these contexts a social capital perspective can usefully guide reflection on current approaches to teacher education and development in the United Kingdom. In part, our interest in social capital emerged from its popularity as a way of re-conceptualizing work in 'the caring professions', but equally it arises from concerns about the way social capital has been defined and used by policy makers (in a rather uncritical Putnam-derived form; see, for example, Putnam 2000) particularly within the agenda of social and educational reform pursued by the previous 'New Labour' administration. While social capital does appear to have real heuristic potential, its practical application within school contexts is only beginning to be explored (McGonigal et al. 2007).

As part of the project we also began to consider how social capital might be working within the relationships and structures of the different school communities where probationer (i.e., newly qualified) teachers were placed, and we were concerned to identify ways in which teacher colleagues, school-based mentors, university tutors and other professionals could be enabled to identify and make use of productive social capital in the formation of early career teachers, and to look at ways in which 'bonding', 'bridging' and 'linking' forms of social capital might be operating. Bonding social capital is characterized by strong bonds among group members, helping people to 'get by'. It is valuable in building a sense of shared identity and security, which is crucial at the early stage of professional development. Bridging social capital then helps people to build relationships with a wider, more varied set of people than those in the immediate family or school environment, for example between students and employers, or teachers and community workers. Bridging social capital helps people to 'get on' and not just to 'get by', and is important in helping employment and career advancement. Linking social capital connects individuals with agencies or services that they would not otherwise access easily. It may help people 'get around', and to make connections with others across differences in status: for example, links between parents of children attending the same school, but from different backgrounds, or between their children. Linking social capital can help teachers connect with parents or children from different social, religious or ethnic backgrounds to their own (Catts and Ozga 2005: 1–2).

In the context of inter/professional working, one can sense that the initial bonding that often takes place for younger or newer staff within working groups can, if relied upon too much as a defence mechanism to cope with the strains involved in new roles and complex work, actually inhibit the useful and necessary bridging between groups of professionals, each group working within their own frameworks of reference to deal with similar community needs, but from a differing perspective. Again, perceived differences in status not only between any professional and his or her 'clients' but between professional groups themselves, can inhibit the formation and generation of linking types of social capital that might help more experienced professionals to move with some understanding and confidence across various professional and conceptual divides.

Briefly, analysing online questionnaires and transcript data from 10 school-based interviews obtained from the focus group involved in the study (24 PGCE primary and secondary beginning teachers), we found bonding capital established: through local authority courses run by advisory staff; from fellow probationers; and from recently qualified teachers, 'knowing they were in the same position last year'. Bridging capital came as new teachers started to make links with other professionals, such as the Area Learning Support Network staff: 'it's good when you're looking for a job, they know your skills, it's like having a friend'. Early in the probationary period school mentors sometimes sought to position their mentees for future job interviews, through giving advice on experiences to highlight and questions to expect. Thus, networks of all kinds proved crucial in the probation year: networks of knowledge; electronic networks (used to share ideas and resources with fellow probationers); and professional networks; as well as friendship groups carried forward from the PGCE year, based mainly on particular connections formed during their shared university tutor group experience.

New teachers' trust in their former university tutor frequently remained strong, and contact with them was sometimes sustained into the probationary year. 'Trust' during this period, however, emerged as a problematic term. In part, trust seemed to be related to reciprocity, as beginning teachers started to feel valued and trusted in turn by school colleagues whose judgement or skill they respected.

What are threshold concepts and what can they teach us?

To illuminate the empirical data on early teacher development from focus groups, questionnaires and semi-structured interviews, we also used the developing theory of threshold concepts. These are now being seen as key conceptual gateways to confident progress in a range of academic disciplines but prior to our study we found no exploration of them in professional contexts. In our project, threshold concepts were explored through the professional events and social relationships in which trouble-some knowledge emerges and is articulated, as well as through the sorts of social capital which can engender and sustain, or else close down, a positive understanding of key concepts for beginning teachers. Since threshold concepts are frequently troublesome or counter-intuitive the need for a clear framework is particularly important for PGCE students engaged in transforming themselves, within a brief intensive period of training, from graduates in a chosen area of subject specialization into effective teachers with a vital wider role within the school and its wider com-munity of parents and families.

Despite the complexities of their new professional work, most of the probationer teachers interviewed as part of the project demonstrated a sustaining 'learned optimism' (McCulloch, Helsby and Knight 2000: 118) through the help of mentors and also through having the security of a relatively stable workplace in which to develop their insights and skills over a school year. But what of 'learned pessimism' and the problems of beginning teachers who get stuck at a particular stage of devel-opment?

Here the theory of 'threshold concepts' and the notion of troublesome knowledge within teaching and learning come into play. Meyer and Land (2003) introduced the term in exploring the idea that within the particular disciplines of higher education there exist 'conceptual gateways' or portals that can open up a student's under-standing of that particular subject in a transformative way. Perceptions are shifted in an irreversible fashion that is unlikely to be forgotten and is difficult to unlearn. Such a perceptual shift is conceptually integrative too in its revelation of the previously hidden interrelatedness of ideas or procedures within a discipline.

Yet these threshold concepts may also be 'troublesome', framing knowledge in a counter-intuitive way; and they are often difficult to teach to students, even intelligent and willing students, who appear to get 'stuck' at a level of conceptual simplicity with regard to a particular 'next step' in learning. For such students the tendency is to accept or create in their minds a simplified version of the concept which their tutors know is preventing them from seeing the full implications or potential perspectives that a deeper understanding of the concept would offer into the discipline concerned. Students may mimic the knowledge without fully possessing it. Such concepts are thus described as liminal or threshold, with some students being halted and becoming 'stuck' at a frontier of knowing. Examples usually given include precedent in law, depreciation in accounting, opportunity cost in economics, entropy in physics, pain in physiology and irony in literary studies (Meyer and Land 2005).

No examples appeared in earlier research in this relatively new field, for the process of learning to teach in primary and secondary schools, nor for the education of teachers. Our project investigated what such concepts might be, and in which contexts they might most usefully be encountered. We also considered whether a better conceptual awareness of such troublesome knowledge might provide a common language for those who share the mentoring of beginning teachers both in universities and schools. The project thus led into areas of liminality and personal growth, and the confusion of the transitions between student and teacher status, and between the pre-professional and professional understandings and behaviours that beginning teachers must learn to negotiate. This transition often begins at the early stages of initial teacher education (ITE) in simple mimicry by the student of how a teacher speaks, dresses or behaves, but with appropriate guidance there should emerge a more mature state of confident knowledge. Through analysis of the discourse of student teachers approaching the end of their ITE studies, we identified nine possible threshold concepts and then set about testing these further using structured interviews with probationer teachers and their mentors.

What empirical evidence do we have about threshold concepts in professional mentoring contexts?

Our original ordering of nine possible threshold concepts (TCs) reflected the formulation of professionalism in GTC Scotland's Standard for Initial Teacher Education (SITE) into: professional knowledge and understanding; professional skills and abilities; and professional values and personal commitment. These three aspects are then articulated in the SITE documentation into 22 benchmark statements and 10 transferable skills. (This group of benchmarks is a reduction from the almost 50 'teaching competences' in prior GTCS documentation that the benchmarks replaced, but are still complex for beginners to comprehend.) These benchmarks are all meant to be achieved in the pre-service year of academic and school placement training and then essentially the same areas of professional competence are to be demonstrated to an enhanced degree during the probation year with the support of a teacher-mentor. We discovered that although our graduates had achieved all the benchmarks by the end of the PGCE year, they still felt that they did not fully understand exactly what some of these benchmarks really involved. We were keen that any TCs we discovered might be usable as an heuristic approach within the current language of professionalism that PGCE students were being inducted into, and not as an additional imposition of terms and ideas in a course where many of them already tend to find too much 'jargon'.

Analysis of the interviews with probationer teachers and their mentors led us to identify the 10 TCs listed in the Appendix to this chapter. These overlapped with but extended the original nine, and we added detail that might act as illustration or elaboration of each of the TCs. This would be useful if these concepts were to be used on Initial Teacher Education (ITE) courses, helping beginning teachers to conceptualize the distinct emphases in the GTCS documents. This might be especially useful in relation to the competence category 'professional values and commitment' which both university tutors and student teachers find difficult to discuss or assess on the basis of sound and secure evidence since the initial school experience (the practicum element) is so fragmented in the PGCE year. Using the framework of TCs might therefore assist in developing student teachers' confidence about their progression through the teacher education experience and its often puzzling terminology.

It could be argued of course (as we have debated amongst ourselves) whether these really are TCs, or merely a reformulation of the existing benchmarks. Against such self-doubts we could mention the positive reaction to the TCs, as currently articulated, of experienced teacher educators, and also of tutors newly seconded from schools. The TCs seem authentic, practical and true to the realities of professional growth in teaching and, being derived from the words and experiences of beginning teachers, they appear to possess an authenticity that gives life to the bureaucratic language of the benchmarks (Cove *et al.* 2008b). Officers from GTC Scotland also showed a positive interest in the study, as did the Society for Educational Studies which had funded the project. Looking back on the research now, we might want to consider whether some of the 10 TCs represent a more significantly transformative threshold than others, and whether further research and investigation is needed into TCs 3, 9 and 10: *language* (learning to talk in ways that children want to listen to and understand); *community* (linking the social and intellectual life of one's own classroom to the homes and streets that children come from and return to); and *professional identity* (finding self-recognition in the confident orchestration of complex skills, rather than in managing to display skill in any one of them).

Researchers in the field of threshold concepts share some of this hesitancy about what exactly these ideas are. The point is sometimes made that the idea of a threshold concept is itself a threshold concept, being hard to grasp in its transformative nature, and also perhaps to distinguish from other fuzzy concepts in the field of education. It is clear that TCs are not 'key concepts', since students who can canter through many of the 'core elements' on the PGCE programme are brought up short by some concepts more than others, and their responses to these areas of difficulty are often very individual. The benchmarks are all key elements to be included in overall course assessment yet not all of them produce the same levels of uncertainty for student teachers. Cousin (2008) draws some parallels between TCs and Vygotsky's conceptualization of the Zone of Proximal Development with its emphasis on the social nature of learning and the transfigured nature of thought that this can bring about. Yet she points out that this falls short of the 'transfiguration of identity' that Meyer, Land and Davies (2006: 21) describe. Threshold concepts can also be related to the work of Lave and Wenger (1991) on situated learning within communities of practice, and with the idea of entering into a discipline, understanding the discourses of the discipline, and being able to interact authentically with peers in the exploration of the implications of particular sets of ideas or practices within that discipline.

This sense of taking on a new identity within a discipline or profession (of becoming an economist, a physicist, a teacher or a social worker) takes us towards the ontological as much as the epistemological. It is true that TCs have so far been more easily identified within the 'hard' disciplines of science, engineering and design than in the humanistic and professional disciplines. Cousin (2008) finds the idea of TCs particularly useful, however, in moving higher education on from a potentially divisive or overly simplistic formulation of 'teacher-centred' versus 'student-centred' learning, by placing subject specialists at the centre of any enquiry about the disciplines they teach. Yet the TC approach is also a humane and transactional one, since the difficulties the student is encountering can only be gauged through interaction with those who are familiar with the concepts concerned.

Atherton, Hadfield and Meyers (2008) describe an international comparative study of beginning teachers in mainly vocational areas of further and higher education, and their revealing attempts to articulate TCs in the subjects they are preparing to teach:

> in post-compulsory education, knowledge is often experienced by learners as inert or irrelevant . . . Since [concepts] are not seen as related, one cannot 'lead to' another, except by association or proximity, nor can an argument be sustained. A corollary is that epistemologically-prioritized or more simply 'cognitive' threshold concepts do not feature much in the experience of learners, unless and until . . . they have engaged with the ontological challenges associated with the transformation of identity implicit in taking on a working role.
>
> (Ibid.: 6)

Some of the TCs suggested by these beginning teachers are revealing. A group who taught literacy and numeracy in prisons identified as the biggest TC for their learners 'the recognition that if a prisoner were to be become literate, he would no longer be excluded from society as hitherto'. Although this might be 'transformative' from the teacher's point of view, the prisoner might well feel more ambivalent, being in a liminal position that could include feelings that he was betraying the socially excluded group of which he was hitherto a member, hence the threshold nature of this concept is clearer. In contrast, those who trained police officers and door managers ('bouncers') identified 'hyper-vigilance' as a key concept, while recognizing that such sensitivity to danger at all times might tip over into paranoia. Those in hospitality and catering suggested 'how to wash one's hands' as a concept – no longer merely an unthinking mundane action, since its effectiveness or otherwise revealed a different perspective on hygiene in the working environment. It had moved beyond a mere fact to be learned in a health and safety module and had become related to the identity issues of taking one's place in a professional group.

Where next in empirical studies on inter/professional working?

Teachers and social workers have different perspectives on the individuals and families that they support in their professional lives. Although the individuals and families may be the same ones, the separate early professional formation that practitioners have undergone, and the ontological changes that have taken place in the course of their training, can develop deep-seated misinterpretations of each other's approaches to a given problem. Beginner practitioners in different professions will approach the same situations – for example, families requiring support – across markedly different thresholds.

Problem-based learning and opportunities for sharing perspectives on practice and values, particularly at the pre-service stage, are easier to propose than to manage within the constraints of time and student understanding at the early stages of their professional formation. Yet to leave it too late is to meet perhaps entrenched attitudes and the negative or 'dark' side of social capital implied in tight professional bonding. One answer is to ensure that in the development and review of professional education programmes, the focus shifts from 'content' to values, attitudes, reflective enquiry and an involvement of the students in broad issues of professional identity. Thus, notions of self, schooling, society, and the development of beliefs and attitudes (including one's own), become crucial to a curriculum that will lead to future inter/professional openness. Learning how others learn can be assisted by understanding how we ourselves learn, and it is here that TCs can offer an illuminating way of exploring both ideas and identities.

This, of course, goes against the grain of what has been current practice in the validation and quality assurance of courses nationally. In education, Scotland shares – although apparently to a less extreme extent – the current close attention in the UK to the acquisition of teacher competences and performative skills. This approach arguably seeks to 'de-politicize' the curriculum and qualifications framework:

> Outcomes-based models, and their accompanying endless taxonomies and lists of desirable learning outcomes and competences, create a vacuum in debate about fundamental goals for desirable cultural and social capital in vocational education and training. This overlooks difficult questions about who is allowed access to these forms of capital, which agencies and individuals are legitimate stakeholders in defining them and whether they are separate or integrated with other subjects.
>
> (Ecclestone 2001: 9)

From a mentoring perspective on professional development, the possibility of the co-construction of knowledge is not addressed within such an approach. Relationships with partners tend to be almost exclusively framed as classroom relationships managed by the teacher, rather than being related to the wider community. Developing professionally is defined in terms of 'learning competences', which require beginning teachers to 'diagnose learning needs', 'plan a learning programme', and 'build a portfolio of evidence', etc.

The competence-based approach is intended to produce a teacher who is skilled in the major roles of teaching and is also able to operate as a 'reflective practitioner'. However, although the principle of reflecting on experience is recognized, it is too often seen as an individual practice. The social capital relations that develop both insight and identity through reflective dialogue with a range of others (we can be mentored in many ways) can be inhibited by too narrow a focus on too broad a range of specific competences. A focus on professional TCs, however, and on any individual's experience of them, may offer an integrative understanding of what might otherwise seem to constitute merely atomized facts or procedures.

For this to happen, much guidance and support for beginner professionals will be needed. A focus on TCs, by its nature, involves the discomfort of uncertainty, whereas professional learners at an early stage of development often seek the comfort of a precision that cannot be sustained in the light of experience. The key place to start in developing a true 'inter/professionality' (an ungainly word for what may well be an awkward procedure, at least initially) is with their mentors and tutors, upon whose confident (inter/)professional perspective their students will need to rely as they grow. Only by students, tutors and mentors listening to each other's histories, by lingering on the thresholds where professional identities that embrace good inter/professional relations are formed and re-formed, might crucial misunderstandings be discerned. And only by pre-service and early-career tutors and mentors providing opportunities to linger and listen will students be supported to understand the different professional discourses and social capital relations needed in good joint-working for the children and young people in their care.

Appendix

1 *Teaching is about learning, both the particular achievements of individual children (often those who have initially presented 'problems' for the beginning teacher) and also the progress made by the class as a whole.*

Teaching comes to be seen as being crucially about structuring or segmenting or pacing the subject content appropriately, in order to meet pupils' needs, increasingly with greater relevance.

There may be a discovery of what assessment is, what its forms and purposes are, how it can shape future teaching and learning, how it can clarify learning purposes and positively affect children's attitudes and awareness.

This concept often involves 'children who make teachers think', and the realization that this is a better working description than 'difficult' or 'troublesome' children.

2 *The same curriculum can be effectively taught in different ways by different teachers across different stretches of time.*

One realizes that it is useless to try to teach too much for children to absorb or retain.

A more confident awareness emerges of the need to pace the curriculum and to judge attainment and understanding over longer stretches of time.

One comes to understand that the rhythm of learning involves peaks and troughs.

3 *Language creates ethos, atmosphere and positive working relationships in the classroom, and beginning teachers can learn how to talk in a way that children listen and respond to.*

This involves a realization of the impact of tone, pitch, pace, emphasis and volume, varied empathetically according to the age, stage, needs and norms of the children being taught.

The impact extends to, and varies within, different contexts beyond the classroom: corridor; playground; sports field; beyond the school gates; and into the local community. (Issues of dialect, accent and solidarity with the community impinge here.)

There is a realization that the teacher's language needs to model for children (and sometimes for parents) helpful patterns of effective thinking and social relationships.

4 *In class and behaviour management, an individual teacher is most effective when contributing to and helping to sustain the whole-school ethos and structures.*

A confident and committed sense develops of the crucial effect of the establishment of classroom norms of behaviour, organization and learned effectiveness (for both probationer teachers and pupils).

Learning to define and to confidently walk the social boundaries between firmness, direction and supportive engagement with young learners is a factor.

Employing discipline strategies appropriately, flexibly and yet consistently in children's eyes helps sustain a positive classroom ethos.

5 *One realizes what makes reflection work, and its importance in learning to teach more insightfully and effectively.*

There is a personalized approach to reflection and where this happens best, and a new awareness of what aids or sustains this.

(Possible sources of reflection are careful observation, conversations about classroom incidents, ideas encountered in current or previous reading, journals, dialogue, networks and thinking time between observation and feedback.)

Apart from learning from critical incidents and colleagues' advice, prompts provided on key developmental areas can promote and support reflection.

There is a realization that effective teachers are thinking much of the time about effective teaching and learning, and planning for this.

6 *One comes to understand one's own role in the mentoring process and what the aim of the mentoring process is.*

There is a conceptual movement from being judged to becoming an active and interactive partner in a developing professional project.

Trust in the mentoring system can be enhanced by a layering of networks of support and advice at varying levels of formality.

There is a realization, achieved through observation, anecdote or the attitude of more experienced colleagues, that success in teaching is variable but that commitment and a positive outlook are nevertheless sustainable and vital.

7 *'Professionalism' comes to be seen as attaining the confidence to make a considered choice about how the curriculum might most effectively be taught by an individual teacher to the learners for whom s/he is most closely responsible, while also accepting the need to monitor such changes in an open and honest manner.*

Effective mentoring can model for beginning teachers this combination of flexibility, reflectiveness and responsibility.

One realizes that imperfection is part of the picture, that learning and teaching will often be successful only in part, but that 'failures' plus reflection can contribute to professional knowledge and growth.

With more experience of working with others in schools professional discourse becomes an aid to precise reflection rather than a barrier to it.

8 *Relationships matter in teaching and learning: recognizing the social dimensions of professional life can make a major difference to a teacher's individual effectiveness in the classroom.*

Taking advice and guidance from others is basically a matter of trust.

There can be negative as well as positive dimensions of teacher networks, especially where there is a lack of active bridging and linking to wider social and professional experience.

Reciprocity and generosity matter in the creation of satisfying professional development: one's contribution and recognition within the community is a source of satisfaction all round.

9 *There is a realization that teaching and learning take place in 'communities' that overlap and affect each other, positively and negatively: home, school and locality can assist or hinder each other's efforts for children.*

Feedback from parents is often a revelation about children or about oneself. (Parents often validate the beginning teacher's effectiveness.)

The impact of whole-school social, celebratory, creative and sporting events comes to balance or symbolize the worth of individual efforts in teaching and learning. (Social capital dimensions of networks, reciprocity and positive bonding and bridging capital have an influence here.)

The teacher's place within the communities of school and locality is realized (with implications regarding norms of dress, speech, behaviour.)

10 *There emerges an energizing sense of 'owning' or 'earning' a professional identity, confidently and realistically understood.*

This involves the integration of particular classroom insights or experiences.

This is often evidenced as a positive skill in the efficient orchestration of a multiple range of educational factors which is rarely lost thereafter.

This is felt to be transformative, at least for this stage of development, and is recognized as such by mentors and other colleagues as well as oneself.

References

Atherton, J., Hadfield, P. and Meyers, R. (2008) 'Threshold concepts in the wild', paper presented at the Threshold Concepts: From Theory to Practice Conference, Queen's University, Kingston, Ontario, 18–20 June 2008. Online. Available at: http://www. bedspce.org.uk/Threshold_Concepts_in_the_Wild.pdf (accessed 18 March 2009).

Catts, R. and Ozga, J. (2005) 'What is social capital and how might it be used in Scotland's schools?', *CES Briefing* 36, Edinburgh: University of Edinburgh.

Cousin, G. (2008) 'Threshold concepts: old wine in new bottles or new forms of transactional critical inquiry?', in R. Land, J. Meyer and J. Smith (eds) *Threshold concepts within the disciplines*, Rotterdam: Sense.

Cove, M., McAdam, J. and McGonigal, J. (2008a) 'Mentoring, teaching and professional transformation', in R. Land, J. Meyer and J. Smith (eds) *Threshold concepts within the disciplines*, Rotterdam: Sense.

—— (2008b) 'Mentoring in the north: new provision, new perspectives?', *Education in the North* 15: 12–22.

Ecclestone, K. (2001) 'Learning in a comfort zone: cultural and social capital in outcome-based assessment regimes', paper presented at the British Educational Research Association Conference, University of Leeds, 13–15 September 2001.

Lave, J. and Wenger, E. (1991) *Situated learning: legitimate peripheral participation*, Cambridge: Cambridge University Press.

McCulloch, G., Helsby G. and Knight, P. (2000) *The politics of professionalism, teachers and the curriculum*, London: Continuum.

McGonigal, J., Doherty, R., Allan, J., Mills, S., Catts, R., Redford, M., McDonald, A., Mott, J. and Buckley, C. (2007) 'Social capital, social inclusion and changing school contexts: a Scottish perspective', *British Journal of Educational Studies* 55: 77–94.

Meyer, J. and Land, R. (2003) 'Threshold concepts and troublesome knowledge: linkages to ways of thinking and practising in the disciplines', in C. Rust (ed.) *Improving student learning theory and practice – ten years on*, Oxford: Oxford Centre for Staff and Learning Development.

—— (2005) 'Threshold concepts and troublesome knowledge (2): epistemological considerations and a conceptual framework for teaching and learning', *Higher Education* 49: 373–88.

Meyer, J., Land, R. and Davies, P. (2006) 'Threshold concepts and troublesome knowledge (4): issues of variation and variability', paper presented at Threshold Concepts Within the Disciplines Symposium, University of Strathclyde, Glasgow, 30 August–1 September 2006.

Putnam, R. D. (2000) *Bowling alone: the collapse and revival of American community*, New York: Simon and Schuster.

Perspectives on identity

Being and becoming a head teacher

Michael Cowie and Megan Crawford

Introduction

This chapter draws on research undertaken in Scotland as part of an International Study of Principal Preparation (ISPP). The study is designed to address the question: How useful are preparation programmes to novice head teachers? The starting point for the study was a shared belief that head teacher preparation is a crucial aspect of school development and progression within the broader remit of children's services, and that programmes of preparation should have positive outcomes for those who participate in them. Four assumptions guide the ISPP:

- good leadership and management can be taught and nurtured;
- the primary purpose of headship is to facilitate effective teaching and learning;
- head teachers' learning needs vary as they progress through their careers;
- cross-cultural perspectives can inform theory and practice.

The overall research objectives for the study are to examine how head teacher preparation programme graduates handle the experience of becoming a head and to consider the relationship between learning outcomes and programme graduates' leadership and management practices as head teachers. A considerable amount of resource is involved in designing, developing and delivering programmes for headship and so it is important to investigate the extent to which engagement with these programmes helps shape the professional lives of those who become head teachers, and how they might develop the skills, confidence and dispositions to work with other professional groups and agencies in an integrated way.

In Scotland, the programme is the Scottish Qualification for Headship (SQH). Although there may be a degree of ambivalence about the immediate practical value of the SQH among heads and deputes who have not engaged with the programme, and a wide perception (again among those who have not participated in the programme) that the programme is too 'academic' (MacBeath *et al.* 2009), no attempt has been made to link the capacities developed in the SQH and the deployment of these capacities in the practice of participants following appointment. Studies of this kind are important because the extent to which preparation relates to what is expected of head teachers and how they behave once they take up post is critical (Walker and Qiam 2006).

Starting in 2006, researchers in the ISPP began to track the experience of first-year heads in a range of countries and contexts. This chapter is based on work in Scotland focused on the experience of a small group of primary school head teachers in the first, second and third years of their appointment (Cowie and Crawford 2007, 2008, 2009a, 2009b).

Background

The backdrop to head teacher preparation is the unrelenting pressure on heads to improve schooling outcomes. Anxieties regarding school underperformance in a competitive global economic environment have intensified the work of head teachers (Grace 1995) and brought political pressure to raise educational standards which may or may not be compatible with the need to work with other professional groups and agencies in an integrated way in the interests of all children (Croxford 2010). The increased demands and complexity of headship over the past two decades are recognized widely. Several studies across the globe point to how head teachers have had to come to terms with heightened expectations, performance management and increasing public accountabilities (Gronn 2003; Mulford 2003; MacBeath 2006; Galton and MacBeath 2007; MacBeath *et al.* 2009), a process Gronn (2003: 147) calls 'greedy work'. These expectations, demands and pressures have changed the nature of headship and given rise to a set of working conditions that many appear to find unattractive. In consequence, the education system in Scotland, in common with systems elsewhere (Gronn 2003; Howson 2005), is finding it difficult to recruit head teachers (MacBeath *et al.* 2009). The integrated children's services agenda and the remodelling and reculturing of the workforce that this presumes imposes a further set of demands on headship.

Another contextual consideration is the linkage of the leadership of the head teacher with school improvement in much of the research literature (Fullan 1992a, 1992b; Hargreaves 1994; Sammons *et al.* 1995; Hallinger and Heck 1996; MacBeath and Mortimore 2001; Leithwood and Rhiel 2003). Although the influence is relatively small, indirect and not fully understood, according to Leithwood and Rhiel (ibid.) the leadership provided by the head has measurable effects on student learning, behind only the effects of the quality of the curriculum and teaching.

Two imperatives overlap when considering head teacher preparation. One relates to succession planning and the need to ensure the quality and development of schools and other services in the interests of all children and the communities that they serve. The second relates to the needs of individuals. From a systems perspective, there is a supply problem with large numbers of vacancies anticipated over the next few years (MacBeath *et al.* 2009). From the perspective of individuals, it is important that people are encouraged to want to do the job and that opportunities are provided to allow teachers to develop confidence in their leadership and management capabilities and to acquire appropriate knowledge, understanding and skills. Both imperatives challenge the principle that people and how they are treated are two of the least significant factors for consideration in schools (Whitaker 1997: 144). The widespread recognition of this is perhaps one reason why the design and delivery of preparation programmes for aspiring head teachers has become a global enterprise (Huber 2004).

What do we know about preparing head teachers?

There may be consensus that the role of the head teacher matters and that preparation is important, but there are considerable disagreements, often philosophical and political, about what kinds of heads are needed, what skills and attributes they need, how they should be trained, and how this should take account of new configurations of schools as extended institutions. There may also be concerns about the quality and relevance of preparation programmes. In the United States, for example, a study claimed to have found weaknesses in the programmes provided by 25 out of 28 university-based programmes describing these as 'little more than a grab-bag of survey courses' (Levine 2005: 28). Although the Levine report relied on outdated data and contained several methodological shortcomings (Young *et al.* 2005), its central finding that many programmes lacked focus and coherence and bore little relation to the realities of managing and leading schools within wider systems could not be ignored.

Despite its limitations, the Levine report challenged everyone involved in head teacher preparation to question the presumption that pre-appointment preparation does any good. While it seems reasonable to assume that programmes of preparation will at least acquaint, if not equip, participants with the attributes required to enable them to deal with the challenges they face on appointment, we cannot be certain that they do. Evaluation of head teacher preparation is problematic, however, and the problems involved should not be underestimated, particularly if preparation is considered in terms of its effects on wider systemic change and school improvement. It is not a straightforward matter to find robust evaluation techniques 'sensitive to the many nuances of behaviour within development processes and capable of measuring intangible outcomes' (Tyson and Ward 2004: 206).

Clearly one single evaluation approach will not get to grips with the complexities involved. It is important therefore to evaluate programmes at different levels. Kirkpatrick (1994) suggests that development programmes should be evaluated in terms of participant perceptions, learning, performance and ultimate impact. Leithwood and Levin (2004) present a helpful framework that outlines the relationship between programmes, leadership practice and student outcomes in six stages ranging through: preparation experiences; participant satisfaction; changes in participants' knowledge, skills and dispositions; changes in practices; changes in classroom conditions; and improved student outcomes.

Too often, it is only the first two stages that are evaluated. The SQH programme, for example, stood up well to intensive scrutiny in a national evaluation (Menter *et al.* 2003) but this evaluation explored the views of recent successful programme graduates and participant satisfaction studies which cannot give us a strong understanding of either the utility or the influence of preparation programmes. With this in mind, the study reported in this chapter explored the perceptions of novice heads regarding the utility of their preparation experience. Although we cannot look at ultimate impact, the perceptions of new heads enabled us to comment on how participation in the SQH programme might influence initial performance.

The preparation context

The politically driven 'competence movement' that emerged in teacher education in the 1990s, is mirrored in head teacher development in Scotland through a national Standard for Headship (SfH) (SEED 2005). The introduction of a Standard for new heads had a massive influence on preparation for headship with the alignment of a professional award, the SQH, and the academic award of a postgraduate diploma. The SQH is therefore a benchmark qualification that is underpinned by the SfH. Programme delivery includes online learning, supported self-study and face-to-face events, but the programme is predominantly workplace based with candidates being required to manage and lead whole-school projects and provide portfolios of evidence substantiating a claim for competence against the Standard supported by a reflective commentary. The SQH takes just over two years to complete. Regional consortia, partnerships of local authorities and universities are licensed to deliver the programme by the General Teaching Council for Scotland (GTCS) following an intensive accreditation process during which partnership arrangements and the programme specification, design and structure are scrutinized in detail.

Attainment of the SfH became mandatory for new head teachers in August 2005. Until 2008 the only means of determining whether an individual attained the SfH was by gaining the SQH. Making attainment mandatory presented the Scottish Executive (the then title of the government in Scotland) with a problem since the numbers completing the programme, particularly from the primary sector, were insufficient to fill the number of posts likely to become vacant over the next decade. In the short term, therefore, local authorities could deem that a person had attained the standard based on her/his experience to date.

However, an alternative route towards attaining the standard has been introduced more recently because, it has been argued, the SQH programme does not meet the needs of all potential applicants (SEED 2006). In the alternative route the intention is that local authorities accept more responsibility for supporting individual participants through increased mentoring and coaching supported by trained and experienced head teachers, with candidates presenting portfolios of evidence to the GTCS to support a claim for competence against the standard, an approach which is in tune with head teacher preparation in England. The universities have no part to play in the alternative route, which raises questions concerning how standards are derived, who is involved in this process (and who is not) and how the process of attaining the standard is controlled. Standards may define, in absolute terms, what is expected of head teachers, but what these developments suggest is that the social and political reality of head teacher preparation is open to differing interpretations.

The research design: three interconnected studies

Looking at head teachers new in post is a developing research area (Crow 2007) but research in this field suggests that the needs of new heads change remarkably quickly in the early years of headship (Day 2003; Holligan *et al.* 2006) and that new heads themselves also change considerably over a short period of time (Weindling 1999). Because the research literature suggests that socialization is a staged process (Aardrts, Jansen and van der Velde 2001; Earley and Weindling 2004), we were also interested in the socialization processes involved. Earley and Weindling (ibid.) describe a two-phase process of socialization for new heads. The first phase involves professional socialization and takes place before appointment through programmes of preparation, first-hand experience derived from current and previous posts and through processes such as observation and modelling. The second phase, organizational socialization, occurs after appointment and it is during this period that personal and professional values, abilities and interpersonal skills seem to be critically important. A three-phase research design was therefore employed in our research. This involved an initial round of interviews after graduates from the programme had been in post for a year (Cowie and Crawford 2009a). Following the first round of interviews, the five heads completed monthly logs over a six-month period (Cowie and Crawford 2008). The third phase consisted of a second round of interviews almost two years later (Cowie and Crawford 2009b). Taken together, the three studies explore the reality of the lives of new heads as reported through interview and reflective logs and consider the extent to which the SQH helped prepare them for the experience of headship.

Phase I

The first interviews were undertaken with a narrative approach in mind. Narrative analysis seemed particularly important because of its focus on the relational, on the individual, the interplay between the individual and the social and the 'reality producing' nature of the interview (Roberts 2002: 15). We wanted to know who our new head teachers were, why they wanted to become head teachers, how they became head teachers, what drives them and how they dealt with their new duties and responsibilities. The idea of storied lives draws on recent developments in social psychology which suggest that self-narrative is an important part of identity formation, and one's sense of self. Head teachers make their own sense of their past, their training and their present by updating their narratives to produce 'coherent narratives of self' (Kearney 2003: 55). Because it stresses the 'lived experience' of individuals, the importance of multiple perspectives, the existence of context-bound, constructed social realities, and the impact of the researcher on the research process (Muller 1999: 223) the narrative approach seemed well suited to an investigation into the early years of headship.

The experiences related by the head teachers were subjected to the 'most explicitly reflexive stage of the analysis process' (Elliot 2005: 158), where the reader reads the text, in a sense, for her/himself, and so we inserted our own selves along with our own background, history and experiences into our analysis of the head teachers' experiences.

The first phase outlined the story of five teachers becoming head teachers, examined their reflections and began to make connections between their experiences. From the narratives it became clear that participation in a formal preparation programme is not the beginning of the story. Without exception, the new heads talked about having been 'talent spotted' and encouraged to accept responsibilities outside the classroom. These development opportunities broadened their outlook and helped develop confidence and self-belief. Secondment, promotion to senior teacher or being asked to take on a temporary acting promoted role was significant for all of the heads, revealing a need to believe that they could become a head before embarking on the SQH, and suggesting that the observation by Day *et al.* (2006) that self-belief influences personal efficacy in teaching, is also true of wanting to move on to headship.

Stronach *et al.* (2002) discuss the construction of professional identities and how professional knowledge is formed in the working through of tensions at different levels of experience, an effect which is reflected in the narratives discussed in phase 1. When asked to talk about aspects of the programme that they found helpful, the new heads could not be pinned down to specifics. Although there was some mention of particular content areas, there was more talk about principles, reflecting on purposes, values and learning needs and about overall approaches to management, integrating theory and practice, developing skills, abilities and confidence. The overall influence appeared not to be related to specific areas of content but to situated and social processes that helped the then aspiring heads to construct their identities as head teachers. Identity formation and learning are closely related in that learning 'implies becoming a different person [which] involves the construction of identity' (Lave and Wenger 1991: 53) and takes place where the social environment and the individual learner intersect. Participation in the SQH appeared to legitimize their role and establish their right to practise leadership and management (Reeves and Forde 2004).

The narratives also suggested that the supportive groups established during the preparation programmes were significant. Working with each other within the preparation programmes also helped develop their professional identities. Through collaborative activity and networking with colleagues a sense of trust developed, allowing the new heads to share and learn with and from each other. In the absence of support from their local authorities, these networks continued beyond the term of the preparation programme and developed into something approaching small communities of practice in which 'a set of common approaches and shared standards that create a basis for action, communication, problem solving, performance, and accountability' was enabled (Wenger, McDermott and Snyder 2002: 38). For some, these enduring networks provided a conduit through which new learning was developed and knowledge was shared. This reciprocity and the value given to this by the new head teachers can also be seen as part of the broader discussion into the creation and operation of human and social capital (Halpern 2005), which has been significant in discussions about the ways in which networks connect professionals (Putnam 1995; Baron, Field and Schuller 2000; Allan, Ozga and Smyth 2009).

There is also a sense in the phase 1 narratives in which the new heads' identities as head teachers were affirmed through gaining the qualification, 'providing a means of entry into a particular social status' (Reeves and Forde 2004: 9). Thus, following Bourdieu (1991), it can be argued that the Standard for Headship constitutes desirable symbolic capital (representational/reputational), the attainment of which increases new head teachers' human capital, while social capital is acquired through the social networks developed as part of the SQH experience. Again drawing on Bourdieu, what seems clear is that the appropriation and use of a social language pertaining to the programme was significant as a medium of power. Reeves and Forde (2004) argue that the power and language of the SQH is particularly influential because it reflects and endorses the privileged managerial discourse of government. In looking at the social processes involved in work-based learning in the context of the SQH, Reeves *et al.* (2003) talk about the authority of the language of the SQH and the power of the standard and how this appeared to be important for SQH participants in reconfiguring their professional identities. In our study, the programme and its related reading also appeared to initiate the new heads into new forms of language and new understandings and helped to validate their new professional identities. Our analysis suggested that the ability to converse within this new discourse developed participants' confidence and belief that they could engage with the demands of the job.

Our overall conclusion was that the new heads were able to assume new identities with relatively high levels of confidence in relation to key aspects of their role, without the 'shock of the new' experienced by new heads found in previous studies in Scotland (Draper and McMichael 1998, 2000) and the decline in confidence levels reported by Earley *et al.* (2002), and that this process of identity configuration was reinforced and confirmed through experience on appointment to headship as the associated concepts were put into practice.

The complexity of contemporary society, however, means that the content of socialization must involve an orientation and openness to 'change in the priorities of the principal's tasks, and change in what constitutes an effective organization' (Crow 2006: 319) as well as change in personal identity. Completion of a year or so in post is only the beginning of a much longer socialization process. Although participation in the SQH helped the novice heads to configure their professional identities and to equip them with the attitudes, skills and behaviours necessary to 'hit the ground running' on appointment, each school has its own accepted norms and values. Not only is there pressure to operate in terms of prevailing orthodoxies as reflected in the 'dialect of managerialism' (Reeves *et al.* 2003), there is also pressure to adapt to the norms of the culture of the new school, and to a lesser extent perhaps the wider community in which it is located. However, socialization processes involve interaction with others and in beginning headship newcomers do more than passively slide into an existing context (Kelchtermans and Ballet 2002). New heads bring with them their own set of values, beliefs and role expectations, although the reality of being a head and developing a new identity may put these to the test (Daresh and Male 2000).

Phase 2

The second phase explored how the new heads handled the 'bumpy ride of reality' (Draper and McMichael 1998: 199) in more detail and reported on outcomes from the log analysis and the themes reflected in the head teachers' comments. The heads were asked to summarize their professional activities each month over a six-month period, note the meetings and events they participated in or attended, and highlight any concerns and successes experienced. They were also invited to identify and describe a significant incident, issue or theme from each month's work and respond to the following questions:

- Who was involved?
- What happened or seems to be happening?
- What was/is your role?
- What decisions did you make? Why? What was the outcome? Was it successful?
- Was there some part of what you did that you would do differently next time? Which part? Why?
- How might you have been prepared to tackle it?
- Was any of your preparation programme useful? If so, how and in what way?

The head teachers were also asked to add other comments which they considered appropriate.

What we found was that although the workload demands were almost overwhelming and the emotional labour (Hochschild 1983) took its toll at times, the heads seemed to cope comfortably with the competing and multifaceted demands. The logs show that much time was taken up with a variety of meetings, in and out of school, often with other professional agencies such as health and social care. This mirrors findings reported by Hobson *et al.* (2002) that much of each day is taken up with a variety of relatively minor but nevertheless important and sometimes quite complex tasks and activities. These demands are challenging because they are relentless and compete for the head's attention. They confirm the significance of well-developed interpersonal skills in headship, the need for head teachers to be able to prioritize and manage time effectively (Holligan *et al.* 2006), and the ability to work effectively with other professionals and agencies, but we found no evidence of significant adjustment difficulties. In contrast to the findings of Earley and Evans (2004) that new heads did not feel prepared for headship despite the development of preparation programmes, in our study the heads were enthusiastic and seemed able to deal confidently with multiple demands. We were able to exemplify this in relation to significant issues or incidents that they responded to in the six-month period.

The incidents or issues reported in the reflective logs were not dissimilar to the problems of early headship in the literature review by Hobson *et al.* (2002) or identified by Holligan *et al.* (2006). Hobson *et al.* found that relatively new heads felt professionally isolated and had problems dealing with several aspects of their newly acquired responsibilities, and Holligan et al. found that novice heads expressed low levels of confidence. The logs in this study also reflect some of the uncertainty that may be characteristic of early headship (Day 2003), but they also suggest that incidents were regarded as challenges and learning opportunities and that they were handled appropriately and with a degree of confidence.

The logs reveal busy schedules, but it would be misleading to characterize the experience of the new heads only in terms of having to deal with a series of big and small problems requiring immediate solutions. The entries reflect the demanding nature of headship, leaving limited space in which to develop educational improvement strategies, but the logs also show that the heads were careful to keep the longer-term strategic perspective in mind when dealing with incidents or issues. For example, entries show them encouraging participation and working to build staff and pupil confidence and capability. The findings in phases 1 and 2 do not suggest that the heads were wholly preoccupied by everyday tasks in the initiation phase, but the novice heads had not begun to focus on school improvement strategies which require educational leadership (Cheung and Walker 2006) and securing staff commitment to improving the quality of learning and teaching (Sackney and Walker 2006).

Phase 3

In the third phase, we continued to focus on how the now 'not so new' heads understood their situation. A second round of interviews in their third (and in one case fourth) year in post afforded the heads an opportunity to reflect upon their experience to date. The focus in phase 3 was on how the new heads had developed and enacted their understanding of leadership. We wanted to know about their sources of satisfaction (and dissatisfaction), about the extent to which their approaches and priorities had changed, about changes they had introduced and about the challenges and tensions encountered. We also explored how they now viewed the job, how they described their leadership styles, the support available to them and how they envisioned their schools' futures.

All were still enjoying the job – most of the time. Satisfaction was gained from making a demonstrable difference, being able to influence lives beyond the scope of the classroom and building effective relationships with parents and the wider community. What was noticeable was that into the second year they began to *lead* as well as *manage*. Without exception the heads referred to initiating 'second order' change (Cuban 1998) aimed at raising improvement capability in the second year, as well as other significant changes that were beginning to produce successful outcomes, and they were proud of what had been achieved so far. Change included: the development of active approaches to learning; ways to increase parental involvement; and the introduction of a more rigorous approach to school self-evaluation. Collaborative working and engaging staff was seen as an important part of enhancing the school's improvement capability.

Although all of the above were a source of personal and professional satisfaction, their knowledge, understanding, personal qualities and interpersonal skills were tested and challenged in different ways. Change often meant movement away from the approach of the previous head. The heads had strategies to deal with any passive resistance, which they compared to the experience of a new teacher being tested by pupils.

The most significant challenge was to develop improvement capability and maintain a strategic focus in the face of pressures from workload and staff, but this strategic aspect was evident – in marked contrast to the first round of interviews. Despite the insistent demands on them, the new heads found time to think strategically and talked about empowering staff and encouraging them to be more confident about accepting responsibility. Determination to retain a strategic focus while managing the multiple and competing demands made on them contributed to the complexity of the job, but although some reported that they had found the demands of the job greater now that the 'honeymoon period' was over, their confidence had increased and they were able to deal with some issues more quickly because such matters had become routinized. Without prompting, the 'not so new' heads talked about and illustrated how the SQH experience had helped develop their knowledge, understanding and interpersonal skills, and provided insight into the complexities of headship in ways that had allowed them to be proactive at a relatively early stage of headship.

The trusting relational networks that had provided support during their engagement with the SQH were still maintained through email and telephone contact and occasional meetings, but the dialogic interactions that had allowed them to share experiences and perspectives and develop new insights and practices had dissipated. The networks had become social networks and fell well short of what can be characterized as communities of practice. While individuals appear still to turn to each other for advice and support, when groups met together they were social occasions, and with few exceptions where participants had 'intellectual discussions again', the heads reported that the meetings did little more than provide 'opportunities for a wee moan and groan'.

Discussion

To what extent, then, did the pre-appointment experience of the new head teachers prepare them for the reality of life as a school head? Our studies were based on self-reported data and our sample size was too small and gender biased to allow generalization or to allow us to come to any definitive conclusions. All the new heads interviewed were women, and women, research indicates, appear to have particular occupational and professional challenges within both their personal lives and practice contexts that affect both how they are viewed and how they view themselves as leaders (Fitzgerald 2003). Our small sample features diverse career pathways that may or may not be reflected in the general head teacher population, but what we can say is that engagement with the SQH appeared to provide grounding in the identity of 'being a head teacher' and that it afforded access to supportive networks that had the potential to become communities of practice.

Our findings in phase 1 suggested that engagement with colleagues and involvement in the SQH programme had helped participants to configure their professional identities as head teachers by exploring and recognizing new ways of being and developing 'new relationships, actions and roles' (Williamson and Robinson 2009: 46). This allowed them to face the challenge of headship with confidence and enabled them to 'hit the ground running'. In the first year they were getting used to 'being a head teacher' and to their school's culture and to new colleagues, and had not begun to engage in improvement strategies or to raise their gaze to the wider remit of headship within the integrated children's services agenda. Clearly, participation in the SQH preparation programme and the completion of a year or so in post represents only part of a longer socialization process, and over the course of the second year the data suggest that heads became more secure in their professional identities. In phase

3, heads highlighted particular aspects of the programme, including experience of academic reading, which had helped broaden their perspectives and enabled them to take a strategic view. What was particularly noticeable in this phase was participants' passion and commitment. In very different school contexts, each individual seemed to be aware of, and able to deal with, pressure to conform to different norms, to have the ability and confidence to initiate significant change and to work with parents, the wider community and other professional groups and agencies. Their emerging professional head teacher identities appeared to be characterized, at least in part, by resilience, increasing self-reliance, an ability to reflect and question, a sense of agency and a commitment to continue to develop their own professional learning and that of the teachers they work with.

However, global discourses concerning modernization, children's workforce remodelling, performance management and improvement are reflected in educational policy in the UK and these discourses have had an impact on professional development (Gleeson and Husbands 2003). The emergence of 'new public management' (NPM) created a complex context of reform and accountability (Clarke and Newman 1997) and the introduction of a Standard for Headship can be seen in terms of an attempt to reconstruct meaning and identity among head teachers, as well as an attempt to control quality and specify outputs, all of which are characteristic of 'new managerialism'.

The SfH, for example, reflects the ambiguous mix of bureaucratic central control that standards represent (Gronn 2003) with a rhetoric of professional autonomy. Analysis of the Standard reveals its opposing narratives and the tensions between underlying values and principles. One narrative is to do with capability and changed ways of working, but the other is about accountability and policy implementation. It can be argued that the need to adhere to a defined standard may encourage aspiring heads to configure their professional identities in ways consistent with the features of 'new managerialism'. Although emphasis is placed on building community, critical thinking, and reflection on practice in the SQH, the programme is located within prevailing orthodoxies. Competence in terms of attaining the standard can be seen as a controlling mechanism and a means of regulating the discourses surrounding what it is that head teachers do. Pressure to conform might conflict with educational ideals (Stevenson 2006) and this locates head teacher preparation within the debate about the nature of contemporary professional identity and places aspiring and new head teachers in a 'complicated nexus between policy, ideology and practice' (Stronach et al. 2002: 109).

It also raises fundamental questions about how headship is conceptualized in the wider context of the design and implementation of integrated children's services, how the leadership and management of head teachers is assessed, the extent to which head teachers are free to act in principled and innovative ways and about the purposes of preparation programmes and who is responsible for their design, development, delivery and accreditation.

One problem with standards is that they give a spurious impression of rationality and precision in defining what competence is and who is certified as 'competent'. This is attractive to politicians, and perhaps goes some way towards explaining why attainment of the SfH is (at least rhetorically) mandatory for all new heads. However, quite how the Standard is interpreted and how aspiring heads demonstrate attainment of the Standard is a matter of debate and within this debate there are arguments about power and about who controls and benefits from the credentializing process.

If, as we have argued, headship, in the current moment of public sector redesign involves complex, practical and interactive processes, then head teachers need higher-order skills, a deep understanding of school and community contexts and cultures, and a firm grasp of theory and relevant research, to enable them to develop frames of reference that can guide their behaviour and decision-making (Bush 1998, 1999). Our study also points to a need to build on the preparation experience of new heads and pay more attention to their support and development needs and to the social-ization processes involved (Walker and Qiam 2006; Crow 2007). The heads in this study reported disappointment at the lack of support provided by their employers following their appointment, and failure by employing authorities to encourage the embryonic communities of practice identified in phase 1 may be a missed opportunity. Communities of practice may also become inhibiting, however, and if networks of new head teachers and children's services leaders are to be encouraged or facilitated, care will need to be taken to ensure that new heads continue to be open to change and encouraged to question accepted notions and assumptions (Crow 2006).

If complexity and change are defining characteristics of contemporary society, then change in what heads do and how they relate to other professional groups, along with changed definitions of effectiveness, are important aspects in relation to socialization (ibid.). Debates surrounding head teacher preparation may reflect fundamental disagreement about what kind of head teachers are needed and what kinds of skills and attributes are required. Universities currently have the dominant role within the consortia responsible for the SQH and are mainly responsible for designing and delivering the programme, which means that SQH participants are encouraged to challenge orthodoxy, to work with others and build communities of practice, to critique the effects of educational and social policies as these impact on schools and their local areas and communities, and to interrogate their own position and perspectives. As postgraduate students, they are required to adopt a critical approach, but independent and critical thinkers may not be required in a system that advocates 'tough, intelligent accountability' (SEED 2004).

References

Aardrts, J., Jansen, P. and van der Velde, M. (2001) 'The breaking in of new employees: effectiveness of socialization tactics and personnel instruments', *The Journal of Management Development* 20: 159–67.

Allan, J., Ozga, J. and Smyth, G. (2009) *Social capital, professionalism and diversity*, Rotterdam: Sense.

Baron, S., Field, J. and Schuller, T. (eds) (2000) *Social capital: critical perspectives*, Oxford: Oxford University Press.

Bourdieu, P. (1991) *Language and symbolic power*, Boston: Harvard University Press.

Bush, T. (1998) 'The National Qualification for Headship: the key to effective school leadership?', *School Leadership and Management* 18: 321–33.

—— (1999) 'Crisis or crossroads? The discipline of educational management in the late 1990s', *Educational Management, Administration and Leadership* 27: 239–40.

Cheung, R. M. B. and Walker, A. (2006) 'Inner worlds and outer limits: the formation of beginning principals in Hong Kong', *Journal of Educational Administration* 44: 389–407.

Clarke, J. and Newman, J. (1997) *The managerial state*, London: Sage.

Cowie, M. and Crawford, M. (2007) 'Principal preparation – still an act of faith?', *School Leadership and Management* 27: 129–46.

—— (2008) '"Being" a new principal in Scotland', *Journal of Educational Administration* 46: 676–89.

—— (2009a) 'No longer the new head teacher: reflections on the value of formal principal preparation', paper presented at the American Educational Research Association Meeting, San Diego, California, April 2009.

—— (2009b) 'Head teacher preparation programmes in England and Scotland: do they make a difference for the first year head?', *School Leadership and Management* 29: 5–21.

Crow, G. (2006) 'Complexity and the beginning principal in the United States: perspectives on socialization', *Journal of Educational Administration* 44: 310–25.

—— (2007) 'The professional and organizational socialization of new English head teachers in school reform contexts', *Educational Management and Administration* 35: 51–71.

Croxford, L. (2010) 'Tensions between the equity and efficiency of schooling: the case of Scotland', *Education Inquiry* 1: 7–22.

Cuban, L. (1998) 'A fundamental puzzle of school reform', *Phi Delta Kappan* 70: 341–4.

Daresh, J. and Male, T. (2000) 'Crossing the border into leadership: experiences of newly appointed British head teachers and American principals', *Educational Management and Administration* 28: 89–101.

Day, C. (2003) 'The changing learning needs of head teachers: building and sustaining effectiveness', in A. Harris, C. Day, D. Hopkins, M. Hadfield, A. Hargreaves and C. Chapman (eds) *Effective leadership for school improvement*, London: Routledge/Falmer.

Day, C., Stobart, G., Sammons, P., Kington, A. and Gu, Q. (2006) *Variations in teachers' work, lives and effectiveness. Research Report 743*, London: Department for Education and Skills.

Draper, J. and McMichael, P. (1998) 'Making sense of primary headship: the surprises awaiting new heads', *School Leadership and Management* 18: 197–211.

—— (2000) 'Contextualising new headship', *School Leadership and Management* 20: 459–73.

Earley, P. and Evans, J. (2004) 'Making a difference? Leadership development for head teachers and deputies – ascertaining the impact of the National College for School Leadership. Educational Management', *Administration and Leadership* 32: 325–38.

Earley, P., Evans, J., Collarbone, P., Gold, A. and Halpin, D. (2002) *Establishing the current state of school leadership in England*, London: Department of Education and Skills.

Earley, P. and Weindling, D. (2004) *Understanding school leadership*, London: Paul Chapman.

Elliott, J. (2005) *Using narrative in social research*, London: Sage.

Fitzgerald, T. (2003) 'Interrogating orthodox voices: gender, ethnicity and educational leadership', *School Leadership and Management* 23: 43–4.

Fullan, M. G. (1992a) *Successful school improvement*, Buckingham: Open University Press.

—— (1992b) *What's worth fighting for in headship?*, Buckingham: Open University Press.

Galton, M. and MacBeath, J. (2007) *Teachers under pressure*, London: Sage.

Gleeson, D. and Husbands, C. (2003) 'Modernizing schooling through performance management: a critical appraisal', *Journal of Education Policy* 18: 499–511.

Grace, G. (1995) *School leadership: beyond management. An essay in policy scholarship*, London: Falmer Press.

Gronn, P. (2003) *The new work of new educational leaders: changing leadership practice in an era of school reform*, London: Paul Chapman.

Hallinger, P. and Heck, R. H. (1996) 'Reassessing the principal's role in school effectiveness', *Education Administration Quarterly* 32: 5–44.

Halpern, D. (2005) *Social capital*, Cambridge: Polity Press.

Hargreaves, A. (1994) *Changing teachers, changing times: teachers' work and culture in the post modern age*, New York: Teachers College Press.

Hobson, A., Brown, E., Ashby, P., Keys, W., Sharp, C. and Benefield, P. (2002) *Issues for early headship. Problems and support strategies: A review of the literature*, London: NFER.

Hochschild, A. R. (1983) *The managed heart: commercialization of human feeling*, Berkeley, CA: University of California Press.

Holligan, C., Menter, I., Hutchings, M. and Walker, M. (2006) 'Becoming a head teacher: the perspectives of new head teachers in 21st century England', *Journal of In-Service Education* 32: 103–22.

Howson, J. (2005) *11th Annual Report 2004/5 for the NAHT and SHA on head teacher vacancies*. Online. Available at: http://www.naht.org.uk. (accessed 3 September 2009).

Huber, S. (2004) *Preparing school leaders for the 21st Century: an international comparison of development programs in 15 countries*, London: Routledge/Falmer.

Kearney, C. (2003) *The monkey's mask; identity, memory, narrative and voice*, London: Trentham.

Kelchtermans, G. and Ballet, K. (2002) 'The micropolitics of teacher induction: a narrative-biographical study on teacher socialization', *Teaching and Teacher Education* 19: 105–20.

Kirkpatrick, D. (1994) *Evaluating training programs: the four levels*, San Francisco: Berret Koehler.

Lave, J. and Wenger, E. (1991) *Situated learning: legitimate peripheral participation*, Cambridge: Cambridge University Press.

Leithwood, K. and Levin, B. (2004) *Approaches to the evaluation of leadership programs and leadership effects*, London: Department for Education and Skills.

Leithwood, K. and Rhiel, C. (2003) 'What we know about successful school leadership', paper presented at the American Educational Research Association Meeting, Chicago, April 2003.

Levine, A. E. (2005) *Educating school leaders. The Education Schools Project*. Online. Available at: http://www.edschools.org (accessed 1 March 2006).

MacBeath, J. (2006) 'The talent enigma', *International Journal of Leadership in Education* 9: 183–204.

MacBeath, J., Gronn, P., Opfer, D., Lowden, K., Forde, C., Cowie, M. and O'Brien, J. (2009) *The recruitment and retention of head teachers in Scotland: a report for the Scottish Government*. Online. Available at: http://www.scotland.gov.uk/Resource/Doc/290701/0089341.pdf (accessed 17 August 2010).

MacBeath, J. and Mortimore, P. (eds) (2001) *Improving school effectiveness*, Buckingham: Open University Press.

Menter, I., Holligan, C. and Mthenjwa, V. with Hair, M. (2003) *Heading for success: evaluation of the Scottish Qualification for Headship*, Paisley: University of Paisley.

Mulford, B. (2003) 'School leaders: changing roles and impact on teacher and school effectiveness', Paris: Education and Training Policy Division, OECD. Online. Available at: http://www.oecd.org/dataoecd/61/61/2635399.pdf (accessed 14 March 2011).

Muller, J. H. (1999) 'Narrative approaches to qualitative research in primary care', in B. F. Crabtree and W. L. Miller (eds) *Doing qualitative research*, London: Sage.

Putnam, R. D. (1995) 'Tuning in, tuning out: the strange disappearance of social capital in America', *Political Science and Politics* 28: 1–20.

Reeves, J. and Forde, C. (2004) 'The social dynamics of changing practice', *Cambridge Journal of Education* 34: 85–102.

Reeves, J., Turner, E., Morris, E. and Forde, C. (2003) 'Culture and concepts of school leadership and management: exploring the impact of CPD on aspiring principals', *School Leadership and Management* 23: 5–24.

Roberts, B. (2002) *Biographical research*, Buckingham: Open University Press.

Sackney, L. and Walker, K. (2006) 'Canadian perspectives on developing principals: their role in developing capacity for learning communities', *Journal of Educational Administration* 44: 341–58.

Sammons, P., Hillman, J. and Mortimore, P. (1995) *Key characteristics of effective schools: a review of school effectiveness research*, London: Office for Standards in Education and the Institute of Education, University of London.

Scottish Executive Education Department (SEED) (2004) *Ambitious excellent schools: our agenda for action*, Edinburgh: Scottish Executive.

—— (2005) *Ambitious, excellent schools. The Standard for Headship*, Edinburgh: Scottish Executive Education Department.

—— (2006) *Achieving the Standard for Headship. Providing choice and alternatives*, Edinburgh: Scottish Executive Education Department.

Stevenson, H. (2006) 'Moving towards, into and through principalship: developing a framework for researching the career trajectories of school leaders', *Journal of Educational Administration* 44: 408–20.

Stronach, I., Corbin, B., McNamara, O., Stark, S. and Warne, T. (2002) 'Towards an uncertain politics of professionalism: teacher and nurse identities in flux', *Journal of Education Policy* 17: 109–38.

Tyson, S. and Ward, P. (2004) 'The use of 360 Degree Feedback Technique in the evaluation of management development', *Management Learning* 35: 205–23.

Walker, A. and Qiam, H. (2006) 'Beginning principals: balancing at the top of the greasy pole', *Journal of Educational Administration* 44: 297–309.

Weindling, D. (1999) 'Stages of headship', in T. Bush, L. Bell, R. Bolam, R. Glatter and P. Ribbins (eds) *Educational management: redefining theory, policy and practice*, London: Paul Chapman.

Wenger, E., McDermott, R. and Snyder, W. (2002) *Cultivating communities of practice: a guide to managing knowledge*, Cambridge, MA: Harvard Business School.

Whitaker, P. (1997) *Primary schools and the future*, Buckingham: Open University Press.

Williamson, Z. and Robinson, G. (2009) '"Challenge", "freedom", "change": an emerging language of activism from Chartered Teachers?', *Professional Development in Education* 35: 42–61.

Young, M. D., Crow, G., Orr, T. and Ogawa, R. (2005) *An educative look at 'Educating School Leaders', UCEA, AERA, and NCPEA leaders respond to Arthur Levine's report on 'Educating School Leaders'*. Online. Available at: http://www.ucea.org (accessed 1 March 2006).

Chapter 8

Professional identities

Developing leaders for inter/professional practice

Gary Crow

Introduction

The nature of educators' work has changed in fundamental ways in the last decade. Although most education still occurs with one teacher and a group of students, the technology of the task and the interactions and demands involved have changed dramatically. Often the various reforms that currently exist to improve student learning and to respond to public accountability mandates ignore these changes in the nature of education. For example, while educational work in our contemporary society requires creativity, ingenuity and complexity, the way educators are being prepared and the images of what is involved in teaching have turned more toward technical competence.

One of the most apparent changes in the nature of educational work is the need to understand education as a process that requires the interaction of a variety of professionals. At the school level, this frequently means a group of individuals with various perspectives, disciplinary knowledge, technical skills and dispositions. Teachers and administrators, in many contexts, are now required to interact with diverse professionals including social workers, psychologists, health care professionals, nutritionists and others to meet the unique needs of individual students. This interaction involves, in part, the interplay of a variety of professional identities that includes values, perspectives, knowledge and skills. Educators are seldom prepared for inter/professional practice, and the development of professional identities that go with these interactions has been largely ignored in much of their preparation.

The purpose of this chapter is to examine the concept of professional identities of school leaders. I hope to encourage a conversation about the importance of professional identity for school leadership practice, in particular the leader's role in inter/professional collaboration. I claim no expertise in the field of identity theory. I have come to this subject more through my research on professional socialization and the frustration with how that socialization, in the case of school leaders, has turned towards the technical and ignored larger issues, such as identity. Thus, this chapter serves as an initiation of an intellectual journey.

To accomplish this, the chapter will first explore the changing nature of work in post-industrial society and the importance of professional identity for one aspect of this work – inter/professional practice. Second, I will examine what I believe is an unfortunate trend in which professional identity is being ignored in favour of a more technical orientation to the role of school leader. Third, I will explore the concept of professional identity – its definitions, importance and development. I will use an empirical study I conducted in England to identify elements of head teachers' socialization that hopefully will contribute to an understanding of the development of professional identity among school leaders. Finally, I will identify implications of the development of professional identity for strengthening inter/professional practice.

The changing nature of work

In the move from industrial to post-industrial society (Bell 1973) the nature of work changed to respond to new demands, new technologies, changing demographics and the increasing importance of knowledge. What some have called the knowledge society (Hargreaves 2004) has emphasized service and knowledge work rather than manufacturing. Hage and Powers (1992) maintain that the fundamental change in the nature of work from the industrial to the post-industrial knowledge society is the move from an emphasis on rationality/linearity to an emphasis on complexity. This move highlights the nature of work as underscoring qualities such as ambiguity, discretion, judgement, imagination and creativity, rather than following a preordained script or set of standard operating procedures of the old scientific management perspective. Hage and Powers (ibid.) identify several characteristics of this emphasis on complexity: the need for individualized responses to solving problems; the importance of human agency; increased substantive complexity; and greater social interaction among roles. Although these changes and features are to some degree only partially apparent in educational roles, there is evidence of their influence on educators' work (Crow 2006a). For example, recent reforms stress the importance of all children learning and, therefore, the need to respond to individual needs with a customized response rather than a one-size-fits-all or teach-to-the-average response. In addition, the demands on teachers and administrators have stressed the importance of individual human agency for the type of ingenuity and creativity needed to develop and implement these customized responses. The nature of knowledge also demands that the work of educators emphasizes substantive complexity, which includes discretion, judgement, imagination and so forth. As I will point out later, not all socialization and evaluation processes in schools adopt this assumption of substantive complexity. Finally, the complexity perspective of post-industrial work emphasizes the increasing importance of interacting with multiple roles to meet the needs of individuals and organizations. Therefore, educators must know how to collaborate with others in these multiple roles that impact student services through the use of interdisciplinary teams and other structures (Crow and Pounder 2000).

This last feature recognizes that the work of educators in general and leaders in particular is not a solo performance. The necessity of customized responses in addition to the profound and changing needs of students in contemporary society reinforced by the knowledge explosion, globalization and demographic changes, demand a network of professional expertise. Multiple professionals, including social workers, psychologists, health care workers and others as well as teachers and administrators must collaborate to develop and provide services for the whole child. To some degree, our understanding of leadership has changed from a heroic, solo performance to more distributed leadership practice in which leadership flows from various parts of the organization, not just the formal leader (Spillane 2006).

This emphasis on inter/professional practice has highlighted the importance of professional identity. In this type of practice, individuals bring their unique knowledge, skills, perspectives and values to bear on developing responses to student needs. These features make up a professional identity. In order to collaborate with other professionals, educators must have a clear sense of their own professional identity and what unique perspectives they bring to the collaboration as well as an identity that understands the importance and role of their own contribution and the contribution of others within the network of professionals.

The professional identity of school leaders, in particular, is critical for the demands of inter/professional practice. Frequently, school administrators are responsible for facilitating this in the school context, by providing resources, enabling group interactions and preparing individuals to interact in productive, effective ways that benefit students.

Trends away from professionalism and towards a technician orientation

In spite of the societal changes in the nature of work that require substantive complexity and inter/professional practice, significant trends are apparent that discourage a professional orientation to work and de-emphasize the development of professional identity among educators. These trends ignore the need for addressing complexity in professional interactions. A professional orientation to work connotes the use of expert knowledge and skills towards ends that go beyond the professional's personal satisfaction (Sullivan 2005). Although there is certainly more to a professional orientation, e.g., language, tools, perspectives, community and autonomy, this focus on values is central, albeit contested today.

Several authors have identified international trends regarding the economy, the workplace and the nature of work that de-emphasize this professional orientation and redefine the meaning of professional work. In terms of the economy, writers describe the 'new capitalism' (Gee 2001; Leicht and Fennell 2001) which has created greater entrepreneurialism, competition and globalization. According to Gee (2001), profits in the new capitalism are made by 'creating new needs and sustaining relationships with customers in which these needs are continuously transformed into ever newer needs' (ibid.: 115). This creates what former US Secretary of Labor Robert Reich (2000: 13) calls the 'age of the terrific deal' and breeds what Leicht and Fennell (2001) refer to as neo-entrepreneurialism which emphasizes competition and deregulation.

These economic conditions and changes have also transformed the workplace. Leicht and Fennell (ibid.: 2–3) identify six workplace changes that affect the nature and status of professionals:

- flatter organizational hierarchies;
- growing use of temporary workers;
- extensive use of subcontracting and outsourcing;
- massive downsizing of the permanent workforce;
- post-unionized bargaining environment; and
- virtual organization.

Leicht and Fennell argue that the effect of several of these workplace changes has been to reduce the importance and autonomy of traditional professions such as law, medicine, academia and teaching. For example, in the US in 2007, over 50 per cent of professors were part-time faculty members – a major increase from 30 per cent in 1975 (AAUP 2011). In medicine, the growth of health maintenance organizations run by managers has reduced significantly the autonomy of doctors. These workplace changes have increased the role of managers who are responsible for assigning, contracting and supervising these temporary workers and subcontracted arrangements.

The workplace changes identified by Leicht and Fennell have, in turn, consequences for the nature of work. Robert Reich (2000) describes three changes: the loss of steady work; the necessity of continuous effort; and widening inequality. Although the current economic recession has contributed to the loss of steady work, the changed characteristics of the workforce described above have also resulted in the loss of long-term employment. Work in many fields has taken on a project-orientation, in which the individual is hired to complete a project and then is let go to find some other project in another company. According to Reich, 'earnings now depend less on formal rank or seniority and more on an employee's value to customers' (ibid.: 99). This requires continuous effort, essentially being 'on call' at all times, which leads to the vanishing border between home and work. Finally, there is furious competition for workers, leading to extremely high salaries at the top, reduced salaries in the middle, and the absence of work at the bottom.

Richard Sennett (1998) identifies other consequences of the new capitalism. When steady work disappears, so does loyalty and a sense of commitment which pertains both to the organization and the employee. Sennett, along with other writers (Putnam 2000), also points to the decrease in a sense of community and a 'corrosion of character' that is evident in contemporary society. These values become victims of the new capitalism, which pervades work life and the sense of contributing beyond one's personal satisfaction or gain.

Other authors document changes in professional work. Sullivan (2005) describes the drift away from the view of the professional as a 'social trustee' to a purveyor of expertise. He refers to this as a move to a 'technical professional' who is more entrepreneurial than collegial and whose focus is more on technical expertise than contribution to larger values and service to the society. Sullivan also laments the loss of vocation or calling of the professional, which is related to the demise of long-term employment and a number of the other trends we have identified.

Leicht and Fennell (2001) note a similar shift in the work and autonomy of professionals versus managers. They provide ample evidence of the growth in numbers and prerogatives of business managers: 'In many of the work settings the control of professional work no longer rests with peers or even the administrative elite of the profession. Instead, control over professional work is vested in managers of the employing organizations' (ibid.: 11). This has reduced the autonomy of professionals over time, so that professionals' work is now subject to external oversight within organizations.

A widespread anti-professionalism is also apparent. Some of this is reinforced by the economic trends, including outsourcing, globalization and other changes which Leicht and Fennell identify. But we must also acknowledge that this anti-professionalism, this loss of faith in the expert, has been reinforced by high-profile ethics violations in large companies, such as Enron and Arthur Andersen.

Hargreaves (2004; Hargreaves and Shirley 2009) sees many of these trends in the educational work arena, especially the shift to emphasize more technical competence. His research in Canada, the US and England identified several consequences to the economic, organizational and work changes previously identified here. These consequences include insecurity, the end of ingenuity and the loss of integrity. He particularly points out the 'compulsive obsession with standardization' (2004: 2) taking place in schools and the development, especially in urban and poor school districts, of 'performance training sects that provide intensive implementation support for teachers but only in relation to highly prescriptive interventions in "basic" areas of the curriculum that demand unquestioning professional compliance' (ibid.: 7). Instead of the professional learning communities, inherent in the traditional notion of a profession, these performance training sects emphasize 'transfer knowledge, imposed requirements, results driven approaches, false certainty, standardized scripts, deference to authority, intensive training, and sects of performance' (ibid.: 184).

In an interesting study in Australia into the professional identity of teachers, Sachs (2001) identifies two discourses around professional identity found in documents and policies: democratic professionalism and managerial professionalism. She notes the development of 'entrepreneurial professionalism', a term used by Menter et al. (1997) to refer to the professional 'who will identify with the efficient, responsible and accountable version of service that is currently promulgated' (Sachs 2001: 155). This focus on the technical leads to what Catherine Casey (1995) refers to as 'designer employees'. Sachs' designation of 'designer teachers' and Peter Gronn's (2003) idea of 'designer-leadership' apply this technical professional idea to educational roles.

School leadership provides a particularly interesting example of this move from professional to technician. Research has confirmed the importance of leadership for student learning and school improvement (Leithwood et al. 2004; Wahlstrom et al. 2010). Leithwood et al. (2004) identify three core elements of successful school leadership: setting direction; developing people; and redesigning the organization. Such an articulation is not of discrete technical competences. Rather, it points to the need for school leaders to draw on values and use creativity and ingenuity to address the complexities of the leadership task. More recently, a growing emphasis on the importance of leadership development can be seen in the literature (Lumby, Crow and Pashiardis 2008). This literature makes the case that the important elements of leadership can be learned, and that to enable professional learning communities to create environments that support student engagement and learning school leaders must develop the knowledge, skills and dispositions. In spite of these understandings and emphases on school leadership and leadership development, the trend is towards a focus on the development of technical skills rather than professional identities. In the US state of Florida, the Department of Education mandated a set of 91 competencies on which universities and school districts must organize coursework and measure outcomes in order to be allowed to prepare aspiring school leaders. These competencies range from legal skills to supervisory skills, but the focus is on specific competencies. For example, one competency states: 'Given a scenario, interpret school advisory committee requirements as identified in State statutes.' Another example: 'Given a school technology plan, assess compliance with State technology goals.' An example of one of the instructional leadership competencies states: 'Given school data, analyze or develop a plan to address statewide requirements for student assessment.' What is glaringly missing is any mention of creativity, imagination, ingenuity, social contribution, civic engagement or indeed of any values beyond legal adherence.

At a larger scale, the adoption by more and more states in the US of the Interstate School Leadership Licensing Standards, as set by the Interstate School Leadership Licensure Consortium (ISLLC), also demonstrates an emphasis on the technical rather than professional. While these standards are not written as competencies nor perhaps originally intended that way, they clearly are being implemented in ways that encourage technical skills and knowledge; again, no mention is made of creativity, ingenuity, imagination or identity (English 2008).

Peter Gronn (2003) examines the standardization inherent in both the ISLLC Standards and the English National Professional Qualification for Headship (NPQH). He notes that the development of national or system-wide standards and correlated assessment processes are the core elements of customizing leader development. One consequence of this customization is the tendency of 'teaching to the test' in leadership development programmes:

> As providers in a highly competitive training market, the temptation for some university programmes to concentrate solely on the learning of model answers and finding ways of making students test proficient, in order to satisfy accreditation and assessment requirements for certification and license, may prove difficult to resist.
>
> (Gronn 2003: 25)

Professional identity

Before moving further to a discussion of the development of professional identity, I want to define identity and discuss various perspectives and dimensions of the concept. Burke and Stets (2009: 114) define role identity as 'the internalized meanings of a role that individuals apply to themselves'. These meanings provide motivation for taking on and enacting a role. Gee (2001: 99) defines identity as the '"kind of person" one is recognized as "being" at a given time and place'. As these definitions suggest, professional identity is not a permanent condition or quality, but is more dynamic and contextual. Gee acknowledges that this does not mean that individuals do not have core identities that are more stable and hold across contexts. O'Connor (2008: 118) maintains that identity has both active and reflective dimensions, 'encompassing both an individual's professional philosophy and their public actions' and that 'professional identities are viewed as the means by which individual teachers negotiate and reflect on the socially situated aspects of their role' (ibid.). Her definition suggests the quality of social negotiation, which we will return to later, that is involved in the development of professional identity.

Wenger (1998, in Sachs 2001: 154) identifies five dimensions of professional identity, including:

- identity as negotiated experiences where we define who we are by the ways we experience ourselves through participation as well as the way we and others reify ourselves;
- identity as community membership where we define who we are by the familiar and the unfamiliar;
- identity as learning trajectory where we define who we are by where we have been and where are going;
- identity as a nexus of multi-membership where we define who we are by the ways we reconcile our various forms of identity into one identity; and
- identity as a relation between the local and the global where we define who we are by negotiating local ways of belonging to broader constellations and manifesting broader styles and discourses.

The literature suggests several dimensions of professional identity that are important in understanding the development and communication of a professional identity. Professional identities are multiple rather than single: an individual is likely to have several professional identities depending on the context and the audience. However, as Lumby and English (2009) acknowledge, individuals struggle with the need to construct a sense of self while maintaining and negotiating these multiple identities. Professional identity is a dynamic rather than a stable concept, i.e., it changes over time depending on factors such as context, experience, life events and so on. Professional identities are context driven at both the macro and micro levels. They are also part of a larger professional culture, which may involve various levels and groups, including the larger professional community (educators), affinity groups (inner-city principals or head teachers who hold to a particular approach to education), organizations (schools and Local Education Authorities [LEAs] where principals or heads are employed), or sub-groups within the organization (elementary principals or heads within a particular district or LEA). Individuals differ in terms of the degree of ambiguity or certainty with which they view their professional identity. At times, perhaps especially at the beginning of a professional career, individuals have more ambiguity about their own identity than at later times. In the same way, perhaps individuals at mid-career experience ambiguity if the requirements of the role change as they have in response to public accountability mandates. Finally, professional identity is developed, and changes, within a negotiated context between the individual and others who view the individual's work. This social negotiation process involves confirming/disconfirming identities and developing trust and social capital with constituents (Scribner and Crow 2010).

The development of professional identity

The literature identifies several factors pertinent to the development of a professional identity. First, as we have said earlier, the formation of professional identity is in part context based and thus it is not surprising that the development of identity is dependent on the specific contexts in which the individual professional works. Gee (2001) notes how important is the recognition by others of professional identity. This identity does not form simply by the individual wishing, assuming or imagining it. Rather, it must be recognized by those who are important in the practice of the profession. This recognition occurs in interactions and dialogue with these other individuals. This is why networking is so critical for professionals and for the development of their professional identity. The professional community contributes to the development of professional identity by recognizing and endorsing the practitioner's view of self as a professional. Second, this process is negotiated. Ibarra (1999: 765) notes that

> socialization is not a unilateral process imposing conformity onto the individual . . . but a negotiated adaptation by which people strive to improve the fit between themselves and their work environment . . . Over time, people adapt aspects of their identity to accommodate role demands and modify role definitions to preserve and enact valued aspects of their identity, attaining a negotiated adaptation to the new situation.

As we have seen, and Ibarra reinforces, professional adaptation and negotiation occurs over time and is more adaptable and mutable in early career stages. Third, Ibarra (1999) suggests that one of the methods individuals use in identity formation is 'trying on' provisional selves. This suggests that professional identity is not an immediately full-blown version of what the identity may become, but rather individuals experiment with different views of themselves as a professional in the negotiation process.

Head teacher socialization

At this point, I use my own work on the socialization of head teachers in England to highlight some issues concerning the development of professional identity of school leaders. The empirical study on which the following highlights are based was not designed specifically to focus on professional identity. Rather, it was intended to examine how new school leaders are socialized. My more recent interest in professional identity has led me to return to this study and others to see what aspects of professional identity I might glean from them in relation to new leader socialization.

My study of the early socialization of primary head teachers in England is based on in-depth interviews and observations over a two year period of a group of four new primary heads in the same LEA (Crow 2006b). I conducted multiple interviews over the two-year period and observed by shadowing these heads in their walks around the school, in faculty meetings, in parent meetings and in board of governors' meetings. Several highlights from these studies regarding the content and methods of socialization seem relevant to an understanding of the development of professional identity among school leaders.

In terms of content, the new head teachers emphasized themes of managerial competence, adjusting to the school environment and self-learning. All the head teachers had significant teaching experience so they entered the headship role with clear instructional leadership expertise. What surprised them, and me, frankly, was the degree to which they emphasized the need to develop managerial competence. For each of the four, taking up the position of head teacher coincided with traumatic school-related events. These events included the firing of the former head teacher, an admission controversy between parents and head teacher that blew up, and a fire that destroyed the school building. In order to respond to these events, as well as to respond to daily needs, they discussed having to develop managerial competence in creating budgets, designing personnel contracts and writing policies. While I would not say their professional identity changed from leader to manager, they did focus attention on developing these managerial competencies.

Their early socialization also involved adjusting to the school environment, primarily through learning to form relationships in order to gather information, implement programmes and create learning environments. They talked a lot about these adjustment processes and the fact that they did not feel prepared to handle them. One could interpret this as their having continually to renegotiate leadership images with school constituents.

Some of the new head teachers' strongest comments came in terms of the self-learning that occurred. These comments about self-learning, I believe, include some especially useful ideas about professional identity. Their self-learning involved several factors including developing self-confidence, learning to be decisive, balancing humanness with not appearing to be unable to cope and developing a hard enough shell to take criticism without letting it affect relationships. One of these topics, self-confidence, is particularly useful in terms of developing professional identity. Self-confidence appears to be a major issue for their socialization, but it is not a uniformly viewed issue. At times, comments about self-confidence related to feeling confident regarding technical skills. However, most of the time self-confidence took on a more personal focus of believing one had made the right decision, affirming one's effectiveness as a leader and asserting a conception of the leadership role. It is also interesting that the head teachers' learning confidence involved both self and school. Self-confidence can mean arriving at certainty about decisions and actions and perhaps even complacency regarding what is necessary in order to lead a school and be viewed as an effective leader. It can also mean the courage to take on controversial issues, such as a more open admissions process, or to take on tasks that are new to the leader. A third understanding of self-confidence can involve believing that 'one has the courage, sense of connectedness, and perspective to motivate others to join in the leadership endeavor' (ibid.: 68). Such is the self-confidence that seems most appropriate for a professional identity that would enhance and contribute to inter/professional collaboration.

Learning to be confident about their schools presented a dilemma for these new head teachers – 'balancing recognition of the school's problems and having confidence that the school can change' (ibid.). Some new heads admitted that when they first came to the school they had major reservations about the quality of the school but over time they developed a stronger sense of confidence in the school's ability to meet the needs of students. This raises the question of whether their image of themselves as leaders, and the school, changed as a result of more effective responses to student needs or whether their view of the school – and of themselves as good leaders – was co-opted by becoming insiders.

The socialization methods these new heads mention that were critical to their learning highlight some of the factors in the development of professional identity I raised earlier. The role of people in the socialization process is central. While these new heads certainly read books, attended training sessions, watched videos and surfed the Internet, their primary socialization occurred in their interaction with individuals outside and inside the school. People helped them develop confidence, reaffirmed and challenged their ideas, complemented their skills, provided alternative conceptions of leadership, modelled skills that new heads did not have, acted as sounding boards, forced them to develop new knowledge and skills and offered expert advice. Mentoring and networking with LEA officials and other more experienced heads certainly helped them develop their sense of self, self-confidence, reassurance in their decisions and so on. Their experience as a deputy with previous heads in other schools also provided learning opportunities, especially in reflecting on leadership styles and approaches. They did not adopt wholesale the style of these previous heads, but clearly the 'shadows of principals past' (Weindling 1992) influenced the leadership images and identities which they considered. Ibarra's (1999) notion of experimenting with provisional selves is similar to the ways in which they use their experiences with these previous heads to reflect on possible alternative conceptions of leadership.

Deputies, teachers, governors, parents and students all contributed in different ways – gaining expertise, affirming or challenging the new head teachers' views of their role, acting as sounding boards and offering advice. The positive and negative tones of their descriptions of these individuals and how they contributed to their learning suggests a negotiation of identity. Some of these informal advisors affirmed their decisions and, perhaps we could infer, their identities, while others challenged their decisions, views, conceptions of leadership and identities. While I did not probe particularly to discover the subtleties of this negotiation process, it is not hard to infer that they were testing out leadership conceptions and negotiating what worked in this school setting. Sometimes these negotiations were particularly painful; for example, in the case of the head whose deputy challenged her more directive approach to instruction. For other heads, the negotiation was more of an affirmation of leadership conceptions, as when a lead teacher and deputy helped the head teacher gain confidence in the rightness of her decisions.

Implications of the development of professional identity for inter/professional practice

An understanding of the development of professional identity is significant for inter/professional practice. The literature discussed and the study of head teachers' socialization described here suggest several implications of the development of professional identity for inter/professional practice.

First, professional identity impacts behaviour. The values and norms that influence how an individual practices a profession are based on a sense of identity. This occurs, according to Sachs (2001: 154), through community: 'Developing a practice requires the formation of a community, whose members can engage with one another and thus acknowledge each other as participant.' Inter/professional collaboration involves the formation of such a community in which the professional identities of individuals are formed, negotiated, changed, recognized, valued and reinforced through trusting interactions with others with similar or different professional identities (Scribner and Crow 2010).

Second, the personal and the professional are tied together through professional identities. O'Connor (2008: 118) notes that in Nias's (1986) study of the professional socialization of teachers she found that they invested 'their sense of self in their work'. For inter/professional practice to be effective, individuals must invest themselves beyond simply attending meetings. The trend toward an entrepreneurial professionalism that Sullivan (2005) decries ignores the sense of self as contributing to a larger whole – a team, an organization, a society.

Third, Feldman (1976) identifies three elements of the content of socialization: learning technical skills; adjusting to the organizational environment; and internalizing the values of the organization/profession. Ibarra (1999: 764) notes 'in assuming new roles, people must not only acquire new skills but also adopt the social norms and rules that govern how they should conduct themselves'. This is why emphasizing technical competencies, as contemporary trends demonstrate, neglects the importance of these values and norms necessary for practising the profession. This is critical in inter/professional collaboration, where not only the technical skills which each individual brings to the team are important, but their values regarding the potential contribution of inter/professional work in addressing students' needs and the norms involved in contributing to a group are critical.

A major element in the development of professional identity is the negotiation of that identity within a context. In the inter/professional practice context, the negotiation process is obvious and critical for the group to recognize the disciplinary knowledge, values and perspectives that different professionals bring to the setting. As mentioned earlier, professional identity is formed not just by the individual imagining themselves in a certain way but the recognition by others of the identity being formed. In the study of head teachers in England this negotiation took place through affirming and reaffirming skills and knowledge, challenging ideas and beliefs, identifying alternative leadership conceptions and providing expert advice. These types of negotiating activities and responses are fundamental to the effectiveness of a community of inter/professional practice.

The development of professional identity for school leaders is critical for the success of inter/professional practice. Instead of a sole focus on technical skills, such as resource management, school leaders must be able to conceive of themselves and have others recognize them as professionals bringing certain values, beliefs and perspectives that can contribute to the inter/professional setting and purposes, and which reinforce the value and practice of inter/professional collaboration. The importance of self-learning, found in the study of head teachers in England, is critical for the development of the professional identity of school leaders especially in these inter/professional settings. For example, developing a sense of confidence based on the contributions of the collaborative team, rather than a self-assured confidence with its attendant heroic role image, is critical for building and maintaining successful teams.

Professional identity is a concept worth studying to understand how it impacts behaviour and is negotiated with others in the school context. It is also significant in leadership development efforts that prepare school leaders in developing role conceptions that enhance inter/professional collaboration rather than only developing technical competence. The complexity in the school environment of leadership work now and in the future demands that the preparation of school leaders reflect this in part by helping leaders develop professional identities that positively impact leadership behaviour.

References

American Association of University Professors (AAUP) (2011) *Trends in faculty status.* Online. Available at: http:/www.aaup2.org/research/Trendsinfacultystatus 2007.pdf (accessed 6 January 2011).

Bell, D. (1973) *The coming of post-industrial society*, New York: Basic Books.

Burke, J. and Stets, J. E. (2009) *Identity theory*, New York: Oxford University Press.

Casey, C. (1995) *Work, self and society: after industrialization*, London: Routledge.

Crow, G. M. (2006a) 'Democracy and educational work in an age of complexity: UCEA Presidential Address', *UCEA Review* 48: 1–5.

—— (2006b) 'The professional and organizational socialization of new English headteachers in school reform contexts', *Educational Management Administration and Leadership* 35: 51–72.

Crow, G. M. and Pounder, D. G. (2000) 'Teacher work groups: context, design, and process', *Educational Administration Quarterly* 36: 216–54.

English, F. W. (2008) *Anatomy of professional practice. Promising research perspectives on educational leadership*, New York: Rowman and Littlefield Education.

Feldman, D. C. (1976) 'A contingency theory of socialization', *Administrative Science Quarterly* 21: 433–52.

Gee, J. P. (2001) 'Identity as an analytic lens for research in education', in W. G. Secada (ed.) *Review of research in education*, Washington, DC: American Educational Research Association.

Gronn, P. (2003) *The new work of educational leaders. Changing leadership practice in an era of school reform*, London: Paul Chapman.

Hage, J. and Powers, C. H. (1992) *Post-industrial lives. Roles and relationships in the 21st century*, Newbury Park, CA: Sage Publishers.

Hargreaves, A. (2004) *Teaching in the knowledge society. Education in the age of insecurity*, New York: Teachers College Press.

Hargreaves, A. and Shirley, D. (2009) *The fourth way. The inspiring future for educational change*, Thousand Oaks, CA: Corwin.

Ibarra, H. (1999) 'Provisional selves: experimenting with image and identity in professional adaptation', *Administration Science Quarterly* 44: 764–91.

Leicht, K. T. and Fennell, M. L. (2001) *Professional work. A sociological approach*, Oxford: Blackwell Publishers.

Leithwood, K., Louis, K. S., Andersen, S. and Wahlstrom, K. (2004) *How leadership influences student learning. Review of research*, Minneapolis, MN: Center for Applied Research, University of Minnesota.

Lumby, J., Crow, G. and Pashiardis, P. (2008) *International handbook on the preparation and development of school leaders*, New York: Routledge.

Lumby, J. and English, F. (2009) 'From simplicism to complexity in leadership identity and preparation: exploring the lineage and dark secrets', *International Journal of Leadership in Education* 12: 95–114.

Menter, I., Muschamp, Y., Nicholls, P., Ozga, J. with Pollard, A. (1997) *Work and identity in the primary school*, Buckingham: Open University Press.

Nias, J. (1986) *Teacher socialization: the individual in the system*, Victoria, Australia: Deakin University Press.

O'Connor, K. E. (2008) '"You choose to care": teachers, emotions and professional identity', *Teaching and Teacher Education* 24:117–26.

Putnam, R. D. (2000) *Bowling alone: the collapse and revival of American community*, New York: Simon and Schuster.

Reich, R. B. (2000) *The future of success. Working and living in the new economy*, New York: Vintage Books.

Sachs, J. (2001) 'Teacher professional identity: competing discourses, competing outcomes', *Journal of Education Policy* 16: 149–61.

Scribner, S. P. and Crow, G. M. (2010) 'Employing professional identities: case study of a high school principal in a reform setting', paper presented at the annual meeting of the University Council for Educational Administration, New Orleans, LA, November 2010.

Sennett, R. (1998) *The corrosion of character. The personal consequences of work in the new capitalism*, New York: W. W. Horton and Company.

Spillane, J. P. (2006) *Distributed leadership*, San Francisco, CA: Jossey-Bass.

Sullivan, W. M. (2005) *Work and integrity. The crisis and promise of professionalism in America* (2nd edition), San Francisco, CA: Jossey-Bass.

Wahlstrom, K. L., Louis, K. S., Leithwood, K. and Anderson, S. E. (2010) *Investigating the links to improved student learning*, Minneapolis, MN: University of Minnesota, Center for Applied Research and Educational Improvement.

Weindling, D. (1992) 'New heads for old: beginning principals in the United Kingdom', in F. W. Parkay and G. E. Hall (eds) *Becoming a principal: the challenges of beginning leadership*, Needham Heights, MA: Allyn and Bacon.

Wenger, R. (1998) *Communities of practice: learning, meaning, and identity*, Cambridge: Cambridge University Press.

Chapter 9

The challenge of articulating a common language

CAT and the socially constituted self

Ian B. Kerr

Introduction

Current models of professional work in Western cultures for a spectrum of problems ranging from the acute psychiatric to more general problems in living or in growing up are currently informed by very varied or 'competing' paradigms which range from the biomedical to the psychological through to the more exclusively socio-economic. Such paradigms may additionally be subject to subversion and misappropriation for political or ideological purposes. Further, current models are rarely able to offer more than the beginning of an adequate, integrated and synthetic account of the contributions and importance of the factors involved, in particular of their developmental dimension. Most of the models employed in Western cultures are furthermore inadequately sensitive to cultural variations worldwide, and indeed within our own broader culture, with regard to the experience of psychosocial distress and disability, the ways in which this is framed, and the ways in which help or support may be sought. Some of these problems may be related to and conceptualized in terms of diminution of *social capital* (see Forbes q.v.) or to the well-recognized effects of socio-economic inequality. There is increasing evidence from at least some models of psychological development and therapy, and from infant psychology (highlighting our biologically based capacity and need for intersubjectivity) that human beings are to a very considerable extent both socially formed and located through a transformative psychological process described by Vygotsky (1978) as 'internalization'. It is argued here that any coherent and robust model of psychological development needs to incorporate a semiotically informed, socio-psychodevelopmental dimension in order adequately to account for individual, and collective, human health and well-being, or conversely, distress and dysfunction.

An important corollary of a socio-cultural conceptualization of the formation of the 'individual' is that there can be no so such thing as purely individual 'psychopathology' but only ever 'socio-psychopathology' and that therefore 'individual' problems cannot be conceptualized or addressed separately from a full consideration of the formative and current social context of which they represent a largely unconscious dynamic fragment. A lack of adequate models to conceptualize 'problems' or issues in a social context may render futile attempts to help or heal 'individuals' and may lead to collusion with underlying societal dysfunction. It may also, importantly, lead to disagreement and stress amongst professionals. However, in a pilot project offering a basic training to a professionally mixed community mental health team using the integrative cognitive-analytic therapy (CAT) model, we have been able to show that acquiring a more coherent, common language acknowledging and describing such 'socio-psychopathology' and its individual expression (in terms of dysfunctional and damaging internalized 'reciprocal roles') can help to focus more clearly and collectively on the task, enable limit setting, facilitate more meaningful communication, increase team cohesion and morale, and reduce stress and 'burn out' (Thompson *et al.* 2008). Further, it is suggested that an internalized psychosocial entity conceptualized as 'subjective communality' may represent a more important dimension of mental health and well-being than the description of more *external* characteristics of a society (collated under the rubric of social capital) and thus merits further exploration. These points are illuminated here by a fictionalized clinical case example.

Background

Both mental health and social work services, as well as various other non-statutory or voluntary agencies for adults and children are, in all Western societies, under increasing pressure to address and offer interventions for a range of problems extending from, for example, acute psychiatric disorder to more general long-term problems in living or in growing up. These problems may be frequently inter-connected and mutually enmeshed although they are most commonly addressed from the perspective of very different or 'competing' paradigms. Indeed some work is informed more by eclectic and idiosyncratic 'approaches' rather than any clear model of theory and practice. Formal models range from the more strictly biomedical, to the psychological, through to the more exclusively socio-economic. Although there is good evidence that a range of factors from the biological through to the socio-cultural are implicated in individual psychological distress and dysfunction (Rutter 2000; Harris 2001; Read *et al.* 2005), most approaches do not adequately integrate these various factors into working models of theory or practice although they often pay lip service to models such as the 'biopsychosocial' as proposed by Engel (1977). Although representing an important advance, Engel's model has also been subject to serious conceptual criticism due to its inability to integrate the various factors discussed and its inability to act as a useful predictive instrument (see McLaren 1998). We have previously argued (Ryle and Kerr 2002; Kerr and Ryle 2005; Kerr, Dent-Brown and Parry 2007) that such models fail either to be adequately socio-psychodevelopmental or dialectical and fail, in particular, to take into account the socio-cultural formation (or deformation) and constitution of the self for which there is increasing recognition and understanding (as discussed below).

This failure is typically compounded by a very Western focus on the individual in mental health and social work approaches, and a failure, for the most part, to recognize that the psychological 'deformation' or problems in living or in growing up experienced by 'individuals' cannot, in fact, be conceived of separately from their psycho-developmental, socio-cultural formation as well as their current context

(Kirmeyer 1989, 2005; Bhui and Bhugra 2007).This is not to say that individuals may not experience and present with often considerable distress and disability and may possess also a sense of unique subjectivity, psychological insight and agency. Indeed the individuals encountered in mental health and social work practice often present with precisely these largely unconscious, internalized social experiences, assumptions and values which may appear, and be, to a large extent 'irrational' and may result in patients or clients appearing to undermine or sabotage efforts to assist them (Leahy 2001). This may be due to, for example, low self-esteem or the operation of internalized 'self-critical' voices. Or they may enact similar critical or hostile patterns towards others. Unsurprisingly, such presentations are very commonly encountered in areas where post-industrial and urban deprivation has been endemic across generations in whole communities. Importantly, the lack of a thoroughgoing model of human experience and motivation results in a rock upon which well-meaning public health initiatives may founder – predicated usually as they are on an assumption of rational, insightful and sensibly motivated individuals. These conceptual limitations continue to prevail despite:

- constructivist or constructionist concepts of the self prevalent within academic sociological discourse (see, for example, Burkitt 1991; Gergen 1994, 1998; Parker 1998; Shotter and Gergen 1989);
- the partial acknowledgement of the importance of social factors within more biomedical approaches (see, for example, Kendell and Zealley 1993);
- the focus in some strands of psychoanalytic (Meares 1998; Mitchell 2000) and systemic thinking (Harari and Bloch 2005) on the internalized relational nature of the psyche; and
- the clear statement of the social formation of self in models such as group analysis (Brown and Zinkin 1994; Dalal 1998; Stacey 2003) and notably in CAT (Ryle and Kerr 2002; Kerr and Ryle 2005).

Implicit in CAT is what we have described previously (Kerr *et al.* 2007) as a 'socio-psychodevelopmental' dimension which, we argue, has considerable implications for models of human development and well-being and for thinking about attempts to intervene in this area. Unless such a dimension is incorporated into coherent and robust models of (collective) development and well-being there exists not only a massive risk of collusion with dysfunctional and reprehensible social process and pathology, but also of perpetuating a system whereby well-meaning professionals inevitably become demoralized, stressed and 'burnt out' (ibid.). This problem, broadly speaking, is recognized by a range of authors within, for example, the tradition of community psychology (e.g., Hagan and Smail 1997; Moos 2008; Orford 2008) who stress the importance of social context in attempts to intervene therapeutically and note the increasingly recognized failure of the idea of 'therapy as technology' (Orford 2008) in addressing more chronic and complex problems. Others from within the critical psychiatry tradition (Ingleby 1989; Summerfield 2001, 2004; Double 2002; Thomas and Bracken 2004) highlight the dangers of inappropriate professionalization of human distress and suffering, particularly in different cultures, or offer trenchant critiques of predominantly biomedical psychiatric practice in the West (Bentall 2009). However, these authors propose neither thoroughgoing, alternative models of psychosocial distress and disability nor means of conceptualizing and addressing them. The issue of the cultural determination and limitations of our Western models of mental health and well-being is, however, important, and ultimately unresolvable, especially given increasing understandings of the socio-cultural formation of human beings as a result of our extraordinary developmental capacity for intersubjectivity and for cultural learning (Bruner 1990, 2005; Rogoff 2003).

Intersubjectivity refers to the predisposition and capacity most humans have from the earliest moments of life to 'tune into' and share the mental states, emotions and motives of others (Trevarthen and Aitken 2001). Our early development is therefore characterized by a complete immersion in, and formation by, the minds of others and the socio-cultural milieu which in turn has shaped them. The importance of this capacity from an evolutionary psychology perspective in contributing to the 'success' of our species as group animals has been stressed by many authors (see, for example, Donald 1991; Stevens and Price 1996). A partial biological basis for this extraordinary capacity (through networks of so called 'mirror neurons') is being gradually clarified (Gallese *et al.* 2004; Rizzolatti and Craighero 2004). Significantly, these networks have been shown to be deficient in severely autistic children who display precisely a difficulty in engaging intersubjectively with the minds and emotions of others. This has led authors such as the cultural psychologist Jerome Bruner to postulate that *Homo sapiens* actually exists effectively as a set of distinct 'sub species' (Bruner 2005), and similarly led Anthony Ryle (personal communication), the creator of CAT, to note aphoristically that 'human beings are biologically predisposed to be socially formed'. An important consequence of these understandings is that there can be no such entity as a self which is universal throughout all cultures, notwithstanding our considerable evolutionarily rooted commonalities, but that socio-culturally formed selves represent sets of distinct and largely irrevocably shaped and constituted entities (cf. Schweder and Bourne 1982; Burman, Gowrisunkur and Sangha 1998; Bhui and Bhugra 2007). Importantly too, therefore, these sets of selves cannot simply be addressed within the conceptual framework of any one model of mental health and well-being such as our current highly individualistic, 'functionalist' but value-laden, Western ones. Nonetheless some models may offer conceptualizations which are more cross-culturally valid than others depending on the extent to which they incorporate understandings of the socio-cultural formation of the self and its collective nature. It should also be noted that many features of urbanized post industrial Western societies, including the breakdown of extended family or communal life, can be argued in themselves to contribute to and represent many of the so-called mental health disorders or social problems which our models and activity purport to address and work with (see, for example, Millon 1993; Fruzzetti, Shenk and Hoffman 2005; Kerr *et al.* 2007). Indeed our attempts to intervene may unwittingly perpetuate and exacerbate them through an inappropriate 'functionalistic' focus on the 'individual' as the origin and locus of any such problems, to the neglect of deeper underlying social causes.

This conceptualization of human development and well-being also moves significantly beyond the important, but more limited, measures of social structure and function addressed by concepts such as 'social capital'. Although this broad but in many ways imprecise concept, notably as popularized in recent years by Putnam (Putnam 2000; and see reviews by Halpern 2005; Arneil 2006; Field 2008), has generated important discussion and insights (including specifically noting suggestive if broad correlations between levels of social capital and mental health; see, for example, Whitley and Mackenzie 2005), it has, by definition, focused rather exclusively on 'external' and measurable features of social or community function such as 'civic engagement', membership of organizations, quantities of social contact, or observable behaviours relating to mutual trust or societal norms. Arguably, too, many of these features arise consequent to and are dependent on deeper socio-economic structures and processes (see Wilkinson and Pickett 2009) as well as dialectically enmeshed psychosocial ones. The concept of social capital has also been criticized for tending to neglect the 'dark side' of community or collective social function and well-being for those excluded from a thriving local community (Field 2008), or for minorities such as ethnic groups or historically-oppressed groups such as women (Arneil 2006), although these issues are broadly acknowledged by Putnam. Above all, the literature on social capital tends, in a rather uncritically Western manner, to refer to society or community as the sum total of a collection of individuals rather than seeing them as merely 'dynamic fragments' of a bigger whole by which they have been formed and within which the meaning and fulfilment of lives continues to be determined and located. This formation includes the psychological 'internalization' of social and cultural meanings and values which represent, importantly, a territory implicitly addressed by the activity of mental health and social work professionals. In this regard, an internalized 'socio-psychodevelopmental' dimension conceived as 'subjective communality' can be seen as, in many ways, much more critical to individual and collective well-being than measures of social capital as currently understood, notwithstanding an obvious relation between them. Such an internalized 'socio-psychodevelopmental' entity is also clearly related to other important features of our societies such as poverty or unemployment (Bruce, Takeuchi and Leaf 1991; Weich and Lewis 1998) or 'relative inequality' as explored by various writers, notably Wilkinson and co-workers (Wilkinson 2005; Marmot and Wilkinson 2006; Wilkinson and Pickett 2009). A further explication of this concept, currently being researched, will be offered below but first a brief overview of the current CAT model of development and psychopathology will be given in order to illuminate subsequent discussion. This will then be illustrated by a brief clinical case summary aiming to substantiate some of these theoretical and practical considerations.

Cognitive-analytic therapy (CAT)

CAT is a still-evolving integrative model of psychological development and therapy which stresses the social and relational formation of the self and its 'psychopathology'. It was initially formulated by Anthony Ryle over a period of several decades but has been further extended both theoretically and clinically by a range of other workers, notably Mikael Leiman in Finland (see Ryle and Kerr 2002; Kerr and Ryle 2005). Although initially representing an attempt to integrate the valid and effective elements of psychoanalytic object relations theory and the then evolving discipline of cognitive therapy (including notably Kelly's [1955] personal construct theory), it has been subsequently further transformed by consideration of Vygotsky's activity theory (Vygotksy 1978; Leiman 1992, 2004; and see Ryle and Kerr 2002), and also notions of a dialogical self deriving from Bakhtin (Holquist 1990; Leiman 1992, 2004) as well as by important developments in infant psychology (Stern 2000; Trevarthen and Aitken 2001; Reddy 2008). This has included findings stressing the actively intersubjective nature (and formation) of developing infants and their predisposition and need for active, playful collaboration and 'companionship' (Trevarthen and Aitken 2001). These findings have influenced CAT concepts of formation of the (highly social) self and, correspondingly, of its 'deformation' or 'psychopathology'. CAT describes early internalized, formative, relational experience in terms of a repertoire of reciprocal roles (RRs), and their associated dialogic voices (Stiles 1997; Leiman 2004) and subsequent habitual coping or 'responsive' (Leiman 2004) behavioural patterns as reciprocal role procedures (RRPs). These are understood to be partly determined by inherited temperamental variation as well as the neuro-biological consequences of early (e.g., traumatic) experience. Common RRs range from at best '*properly cared for–properly caring for*', for example, through to, at another extreme, '*neglected and abused–neglecting and abusing*'.

CAT adopts a fundamentally relational focus, therefore, and stresses the importance of the transformative and mutative psychological 'internalization' within a developing 'individual' of surrounding social structures and conditions, and of semiotically mediated interpersonal experience. The outcome of this process is an 'individual' who is socially formed and constituted by developmental interpersonal experience and cultural values and whose very sense of subjective self, relations with others, behaviour and values are socially determined and relative, and are for the most part unconscious. A very brief quote from the philosopher of the 'dialogic' self, Bakhtin, whose work has been an important recent influence on CAT, may give a flavour of this:

> a person has no internal sovereign territory; s/he is wholly and always on the boundary; looking into her/himself, s/he looks into the eyes of another – or with the eyes of another.
>
> (Bakhtin 1984: 287–8)

A well-known quote from Vygotsky may also give a sense of the concept of inter-nalization, stressing the *inter*personal origins of *intra*personal 'activity' through a mutative and transformative process:

> Any function in a child's cultural development appears twice, or on two planes. First it appears on the social plane and then on the psychological plane. First it appears between people as an interpsychological category and then within the child as an intrapsychological category. This is equally true with regard to volun-tary attention, logical memory, the formation of concepts and the development of volition. We may consider this position as a law in the full sense of the word,

but it goes without saying that internalization transforms the process itself and changes its structure and functions. Social relations or relations among people genetically underlie all higher functions and their relationships.

(Vygotsky 1978: 163)

(See Cox and Lightfoot [1997] for further discussion and accounts of empirically supported elaborations of this theory.) An important corollary of the process of internalization, understood in this Vygotskian sense is that, as noted above, although it is an individual who experiences and presents with distress and disability, there is in an important sense no such thing as individual 'psychopathology', but only 'socio-psychopathology'. This statement, which is probably, to most contemporary, post-Cartesian, Western sensibilities, largely counter-intuitive, will be further elaborated below.

CAT focuses on the internalized social and relational origins of a patient's problems (repertoire of RRs and RRPs) and offers a means of addressing these both in general but also as they may be enacted within the therapeutic relationship. This work is aided by the use of summary 'reformulation' letters and maps which are conceived of in the language of Vygotsky as 'psychological tools'.

The professional or therapeutic relationship and its setting is, for many patients and social work clients, frequently experienced as perplexing, frustrating and provocative, and often leads to coping in habitual ways which may be experienced or construed by professionals as 'difficult' or 'hard to help' (Kerr 1999; Leahy 2001; Ryle and Kerr 2002; Kerr and Leighton 2008). Frequently, frustrated knee-jerk 'reactions' by professionals may all too easily then result in (collusive) rejection and annoyance – thereby often compounding familiar early formative experiences for patients and clients (Kerr *et al.* 2007) and effectively representing collusion with the patient or client's repertoire of RRs. Therapeutic work in CAT focuses on the collaborative description of the formative, often largely unconscious, RRs and the coping patterns (RRPs – including associated core beliefs, dialogic voices [Holquist 1990] and emotional states) and, importantly, their consequences (usually reinforcing initial formative experiences in 'vicious cycles'), and then on attempting to help patients to try things differently in the context of a more benign and facilitating relationship. However, the latter, although important, is rarely in itself enough and indeed may constitute colluding with a '*needy victim–sympathetic carer*' RR, for example, to the neglect of other more 'difficult' RR enactments, like 'abusing' or 'self-sabotaging'. It is important to be aware of all of these in professional work – especially given that such collusion may perpetuate or unwittingly exacerbate the difficulties with which a patient or client presents (an example is discussed in the case below).

Implicit also in these reformulations, in addition to their powerfully acknowledging a personal narrative, is a depiction of a particular socio-cultural formative and current context which is usually beyond the remit or power of mental health professionals, for example, to address or modify. Nonetheless, such cultural micro-mapping may be important in acknowledging and noting the impact of such influences and how they may affect attempts to offer therapy or social assistance. In this respect the process has obvious parallels and overlaps with the 'social power mapping' described by Hagan and Smail (1997). Arguably the CAT approach offers a clearer and more effective means of conceptualizing and dealing with the risk of collusion either directly with a patient or with a professional care group by means of techniques such as contextual ('systemic') reformulation or mapping (see Figures 9.1–3 below, and Kerr 1999; Ryle and Kerr 2002). Indeed, increasingly, in a move away from standard individual therapy or case work, CAT is being used to inform systemic consultancy work whether clinical or organizational. We have argued that such mapping is in fact always applicable, even if not immediately obvious, with every 'individual' treated or cared for by our services.

A further implication of the CAT model and of these understandings is that ultimately therapy or social assistance may only, or best, be achieved by engaging the ownership, support and participation of a 'broader community' at large – as opposed to professionalizing a response inappropriately as has tended to occur within, for example, the Improving Access to Psychological Therapies[1] initiative in England and comparable initiatives in Scotland[2] and elsewhere – notwithstanding that specialist understandings and expertise may be required to underpin or support mental health and well-being initiatives overall. Such approaches are historically partly embodied in the therapeutic community tradition (Kennard 1999) although arguably this has lacked a coherent theoretical basis beyond embodying (important) ideals such as 'democratization', 'communalism', 'reality confrontation' and so forth (Kerr 2000). But to move towards this broader community approach a major paradigm shift is required, which our services and our society as a whole will need to address, implement and evaluate. At the least, in routine day-to-day work, a coherent model of the socially constituted self can enable better communication and lessen professional stress. We have previously described a largely successful pilot project which offered an intensive skills-level training in CAT to a mixed professional group in an attempt to achieve this (Thompson et al. 2008). An example of this approach to thinking about treatment is given below. Contextual and social factors, both formative and current, are highlighted along with the challenges implicit to our ways of working. The example also highlights the need for coherent, culturally sensitive and robust models of human development, mental health and well-being.

A socio-psychodevelopmental dimension and internalized 'subjective communality'

From the foregoing CAT-informed considerations the view is taken here that a fundamentally important aspect of what 'individuals' in our culture and society present with, and what we as professionals address, is the (mutative) internalization of formative socio-cultural experience and values. This includes broader social conditions and norms which may also include, for example, religious affiliations or cultural values. In particular, an important dimension of the psychosocial internalized world of patients and clients is that representing what Kerr, Ryle and Abernathy (work in progress) have called 'subjective communality'. This is conceived as representing the formative internalization of a sense of collective identity, meaning and purpose, a sense of mutual support and trust, and a sense of acknowledgement and appreciation of personal experience and narrative. Initial clinical impressions suggest that this represents an important dimension of mental health and well-being and appears to correlate with conventional measures of mental health problems. Furthermore, it undoubtedly limits and determines the long-term outcome of any intervention whether primarily of a psychological, pharmacological or social nature. This contextual limitation is in fact well recognized broadly in terms of outcome and recovery from, and also ætiology of, for example, post-traumatic disorders (Summerfield 2001, 2004) or even psychotic disorders (Warner 1994; Read *et al.* 2005). We argue that this construct represents a more meaningful, immediately proximate and important dimension for our work which more genuinely represents the internalization of the quality of social and community life than that offered by the notion of social capital. Social capital represents, we argue, more of a psychosocial epiphenomenon – although there are obvious commonalities and overlaps with some features of 'subjective communality' such as levels of mutual trust. Implicit in the construct of subjective communality too, however, is a paradigmatic challenge to conventional Western notions by suggesting that the individual constitutes a dynamic fragment of a social whole both in formation and context, and cannot be considered apart from this. It also challenges the demonstrably illusory but deeply ingrained Western (particularly North American) belief that meaning and fulfilment in life can somehow be achieved on a purely individual basis (Ryle and Kerr 2002). A similar argument has been propounded by authors such as James (2007, 2008), although arguably he does so from a more individualistic perspective and does not move to consider the further implications of a socially constituted self. This shift represents conceptually a reversion in many ways to more generally accepted but unconscious understandings of our social psychology from earlier (collective) ways of life in our evolutionary history. This understanding frequently represents in our experience (Kerr and Ryle 2005) a major stumbling block at an experiential level for both trainees in this model of psychotherapy but also more generally for professional colleagues of various backgrounds – not to mention the general public.

A fictionalised case showing extended CAT-based 'contextual' reformulation

JIM – 'NOT UP TO IT'

Jim was a young man in his early twenties who had been referred for assessment and possible treatment to a therapeutic community by a despairing probation service following his release from prison where he had been serving a sentence for a serious assault. Whilst in prison he had been diagnosed with a probable mixed antisocial and borderline type personality disorder and had seen a psychologist for a course of cognitive behavioural therapy, but he had dropped out saying it just wasn't relevant. However, it was felt that there were significant psychological 'issues' underlying his difficulties and he was willing to be referred.

Jim's background included an upbringing in a deprived inner-city area in a highly dysfunctional family (for implications of this see Millon 1993; Fruzzetti *et al.* 2005) where both parents drank heavily and argued constantly and his father in particular teased, taunted and beat him frequently, saying he was worthless and useless. He had learned early on to keep things to himself and to try to cope alone. He had done poorly at school where he had overall felt ignored and rejected by staff although he had been a talented sportsman and had a trial for a well-known local football club. However he was dropped by them due to his increasing alcohol and drug misuse. He had several brief relationships, all ultimately characterized by arguments and fights. He had a son by one of these girlfriends with whom he had little contact at that time. Jim was currently living back home with his by now elderly mother.

At assessment, he came over as 'touchy', 'wary' and rather 'paranoid' although he also presented with obvious distress and unhappiness about his situation and stated that he really wanted to 'give it a go', partly for his son for whom he 'wanted to do better'. Despite considerable misgivings about his motivation and capacity to engage he was offered a place in a therapeutic community which he took up. However, his progress in settling in was slow and characterized by continued wariness and a pattern of withdrawing from groups and activities when questioned or challenged, or of getting into arguments. The community found him hard to support. However, he continued to express a determination to 'stick' with it although it became clear that he struggled with the idea that treatment was not a passive process but something with which he would need to engage actively. His presentation elicited different reactions from the community, with some (mostly female) members often being sympathetic and concerned for him whilst some others were resentful or actually afraid. Finally, however, he became involved in a heated argument in a group session during which he stood up and threatened another (male) group member although he was dissuaded from acting. He then threw a chair across the room, stormed off and left the building. The community heard some time later that he had been arrested following a further fight in a pub and was back in prison. Reactions to these events were varied and included the views that he 'hadn't been really motivated', 'was taking the piss', 'was dangerous', was 'psychologically badly damaged', was 'projecting his anger onto the community', was 'doing his best', 'needed anger management' and, overall, that he was 'not up to it'. Some months later a letter arrived from Jim in prison saying that he had been thinking about his experiences and that he felt he had gained something from his brief time in the community and that he had some better idea of what 'pushed his buttons and why' and that maybe at some time in the future he would like to give it another go.

Overall, Jim's story illustrates a sadly not uncommon experience in contemporary Western society (and also in others) where adverse early interpersonal experience as well as its social context and cultural values are internalized in an individual in a profoundly damaging way, leading to a trajectory of ever worsening and self-perpetuating difficulties for which, all too often, an individual is 'blamed'. These for Jim culminated in an unhelpful but inevitable detention within the prison system and the diagnosis of a formal mental disorder. Both of these occurrences can be seen to represent also the workings of a dysfunctional social system. Tragically his very difficulties led to misunderstandings and rejection at school, by the prison and pro-bation service and then later by a therapeutic community. None of their approaches was adequate to engage and help such an individual, although some members of these institutions obviously felt concern and also impotence in the face of these ultimately systemic difficulties. Incidentally, and importantly, Jim's sense of internalized 'subjective communality' would clearly have been very low (as can be inferred from Figures 9.1–3). Figures 9.1–3 also illustrate how, critically, when he felt humiliated he could explode with 'justified' rage – a very common and well-documented dynamic in violent acts (especially among males) in those who end up in prison (Gilligan 2000). Critically, services lacked a clear and robust model with which to describe these experiences and their consequences. The series of diagrams in Figures 9.1–3 represents an attempt to outline and describe from a CAT perspective in a non-judgemental fashion these experiences and their consequences and also systemic pressures and reactions. On this basis, at some point in Jim's story this perspective might arguably have improved understandings and enabled more effective action to be taken in a more 'joined-up' way by the various professionals and others involved. On a more positive note, Jim had clearly managed to retain some sense of hope and concern for others (notably his son). This might possibly enable him at some point in the future to seek appropriate help again and get off the pathway on which he has found himself, although the statistics for such outcomes for those who find themselves in his position are not currently encouraging. Finally, rather than asking whether Jim was 'up to it', the question might better be posed as to whether our collective understandings and systems are 'up to it'.

CAT Map: 'Jim' – key formative reciprocal roles

neglecting, unhearing
'doing down', abusing

neglected, unheard
'done down', abused

Figure 9.1 Diagram showing formative (compound) reciprocal roles (RRs) for Jim.

CAT Map: 'Jim' – key RRs and coping enactments – reciprocal role procedures

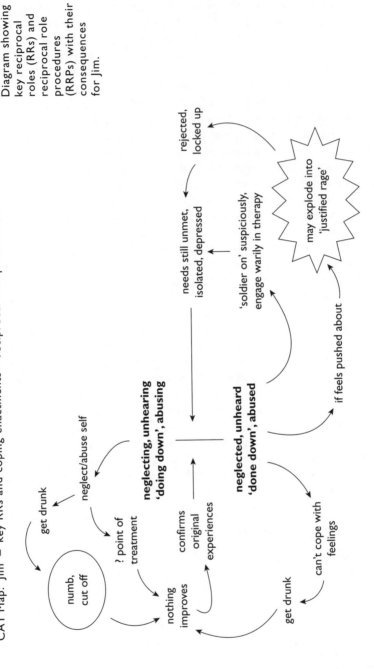

Figure 9.2
Diagram showing key reciprocal roles (RRs) and reciprocal role procedures (RRPs) with their consequences for Jim.

CAT Map: 'Jim' – including systemic reciprocal role reactions

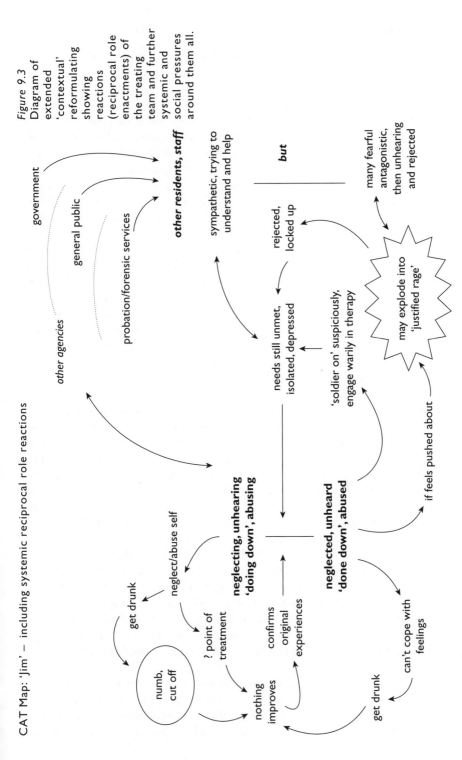

Figure 9.3
Diagram of
extended
'contextual'
reformulating
showing
reactions
(reciprocal role
enactments) of
the treating
team and further
systemic and
social pressures
around them all.

Conclusions

The 'caring professions', including mental health and social work both in general and also for young people, face major and increasing challenges and pressures to address an apparently inexorable rising tide of problems which may be ultimately largely attributable to societal dysfunction (Wilkinson 2005; James 2007, 2008; Kerr *et al.* 2007; Wilkinson and Pickett 2009). This pressure is undoubtedly due in part to an increasing acceptance and destigmatization of mental health and social problems. However, the location of these problems 'in' the individual and their 'functionalistic' attribution can be argued to represent, rather paradoxically, a version of Marcuse's (1964) notion of 'repressive desublimation' in that this acceptance and focus can be seen to distract from the need to address the 'bigger picture' and ultimate (socio-psychodevelopmental) causes of these problems, as argued here. Whatever their status, such problems have contributed to a demand for services and solutions from the general public as well as politicians and agencies such as the judicial system. But the challenge of addressing these problems is compounded by the absence of coherent and integrated models with which to understand and address them. Instead, there exists a range of models with different perspectives on the nature of such problems and of their solutions. Above all, there exists a very Western pressure and tendency to conceive of mental health and social problems as being somehow a 'functional' technical problem located within or around the individual. This applies whether the difficulties are conceived in terms of abnormal genetics or biochemistry, psychological structures or social circumstances. All of these points are illustrated to some extent by the case discussed above.

Understandings and literature such as those generated in the social capital tradition have contributed stimulating insights and discussion on this topic. Nonetheless these approaches remain essentially focused on more external features of society and as such represent epiphenomena related to deeper underlying determinative structures – including socio-cultural factors. It is argued here that an adequate model acknow-ledging the socially constituted self must ultimately bridge disciplines; for example, in a process Wilson (1998) terms 'consilience' (the interlocking of causal explana-tions across different intellectual disciplines). Such models must also offer a coherent integrative and synthetic account of the various factors which contribute to the formation or deformation of the individual and offer, predictively, suggestions for practical action. Authors such as James (2007, 2008) and Wilkinson (2005; Wilkinson and Pickett 2009) indeed attempt to do so from a very complementary perspective to that offered here. However we (Kerr *et al.* 2007) have also suggested that, given emerging understandings regarding the radically social formation of the self through mechanisms such as intersubjectivity, following, for example, Vygotsky, it is also evident that in fact there is no such thing as individual psychopathology but only ever 'socio-psychopathology'.

This position contains a clear acknowledgement that for the most part the major determinants of our individual and collective mental health and well-being are socio-cultural and socio-economic and incorporate both the consequences of aspects of our collective life such as poverty or especially inequality (Bruce *et al.* 1991; Weich and

Lewis 1998; Wilkinson 2005; Wilkinson and Pickett 2009) but also culturally relative and variable values and norms. Collectively these cannot be ultimately incorporated into one standard universal model of mental health and well-being despite implicit Western aspirations to do so. It is suggested that, although such (culturally relative) integrative models are far from complete or fully worked out, we can begin to suggest what their components might look like – notwithstanding that we still do not have, for example, means of assessing fully the genetic background of an individual, or a fully meaningful account of their upbringing and early interpersonal experience, or of a current life situation as experienced by an individual – never mind their developmental and dialectical interactions (see also, for example, Rutter 2000; Harris 2001; Bolton and Hill 2003). Such models, however, even in their early formulations, should and can (Thompson *et al.* 2008) be taught routinely, we argue, ideally during initial professional pre-registration training, to a whole range of professionals from psychiatry and nursing through to social work and other statutory services such as the judicial system or education. Models that take account of the socially constituted self need also to be translated into the public domain and democratized in order that these emerging fundamental understandings of the constituents of our (collective) health and well-being can be addressed and acted upon along with more commonly accepted understandings in public health of issues such as sanitation, hygiene or diet. In particular, such a model of mental health and well-being represents a major challenge to, currently, highly individualized approaches to and assumptions about this territory as well as about meaning and fulfilment in life in general. Many of the interventions which will be required to improve mental health and well-being overall in our societies will need to occur at a broader socio-economic level.

Finally, it is suggested that an entity here conceptualized as 'subjective communality', representing an internalized psychosocial dimension within patients and clients in our public services, may prove to be much more important than the external functional features of a society addressed by other social theory such as social capital. A conceptualization of subjective communality also complements emerging understandings that mental health and well-being cannot be an individual 'achievement' but are rather rooted and located in our collective life. It is consistent also with the assertion that, ultimately, active participation in society at large will in the end be critically important in owning, acknowledging and addressing (collective) mental health and well-being. Above all there is a continuing need for cross-disciplinary bridging and joint building of new conceptual models without which we will continue to operate in professional 'bunkers' – each in effect ignoring what the other is doing, undermining our effectiveness and frequently unwittingly colluding in the construction of underlying sociopathogenic causes.

Acknowledgements

Much of the material presented in this chapter represents and draws on previous work undertaken by numerous colleagues and collaborators, notably Dr Anthony Ryle.

Notes

1   http://www.iapt.nhs.uk/.
2   http://www.nes.scot.nhs.uk/mentalhealth/.

References

Arneil, B. (2006) *Diverse communities: the problem with social capital*, Cambridge: Cambridge University Press.
Bakhtin, M. M. (1984) *Problems of Dostoevsky's poetics*, Minneapolis, MN: University of Minnesota Press.
Bentall, R. (2009) *Doctoring the mind: why psychiatric treatments fail*, London: Penguin.
Bhui, K. and Bhugra, D. (eds) (2007) *Culture and mental health*, London: Hodder Arnold.
Bolton, D. and Hill, J. (2003) *Mind, meaning and mental disorder. The nature of causal explanation in psychology and psychiatry*, Oxford: Oxford University Press.
Brown, D. and Zinkin, L. (1994) *The psyche and the social world – developments in group analytic theory*, London: Routledge.
Bruce, M. L., Takeuchi, D. T. and Leaf, P. J. (1991) 'Poverty and psychiatric status. Longitudinal evidence from the New Haven Epidemiologic Catchment Area Study', *Archives of General Psychiatry* 48: 470–4.
Bruner, J. (1990) *Acts of meaning*, Cambridge, MA: Harvard University Press.
—— (2005) '*Homo sapiens*, a localised species', *Behavioral and Brain Sciences* 28: 694–5.
Burkitt, I. (1991) *Social selves: theories of the social formation of personality*, London: Sage Publications.
Burman, E., Gowrisunkur, J. and Sangha, K. (1998) 'Conceptualizing cultural and gendered identities in psychological therapies', *The European Journal of Psychotherapy, Counselling and Health* 1: 231–56.
Cox, B. D. and Lightfoot, C. (eds) (1997) *Sociogenetic perspectives on internalization*, Mahwah, NJ: Lawrence Erlbaum Associates.
Dalal, F. (1998) *Taking the group seriously*, London: Jessica Kingsley.
Donald, M. (1991) *Origins of the modern mind: three stages in the evolution of culture and cognition*, Cambridge MA: Harvard University Press.
Double, D. (2002) 'The limits of psychiatry', *British Medical Journal* 324: 900–04.
Engel, G. L. (1977) 'The need for a new medical model: a challenge for biomedicine', *Science* 196: 129–36.
Field, J. (2008) *Social capital*, London: Routledge.
Fruzzetti, A. E., Shenk, C. and Hoffman, P. D. (2005) 'Family interaction and the development of borderline personality disorder: a transactional model', *Development and Psychopathology* 17:1007–30.
Gallese, V., Keysers, C. and Rizzolatti, G. (2004) 'A unifying view of the basis of social cognition', *Trends in Cognitive Sciences* 8: 396–403.
Gergen, K. (1994) 'Exploring the post modern: perils or potentials?', *American Psychologist* 49: 412–16.
—— (1998) *An invitation to social constructionism*, London: Sage.
Gilligan, J. (2000) *Violence: reflections on our deadliest epidemic*, London: Jessica Kingsley.
Hagan, T. and Smail, D. (1997) 'Power-mapping 1. Background and basic methodology', *Journal of Community and Applied Social Psychology* 7: 257–67.
Halpern, D. (2005) *Social capital*, Cambridge: Polity Press.
Harari, E. and Bloch, S. (2005) 'Family therapy', in S. Bloch (ed.) *An introduction to the psychotherapies*, Oxford: Oxford University Press.

Harris, T. (2001) 'The psychosocial origins of depression', *British Medical Bulletin* 57: 17–32.

Holquist, M. (1990) *Dialogism*, London: Routledge.

Ingleby, D. (1989) 'Critical psychology in relation to political repression and violence', *International Journal of Mental Health* 17: 16–28.

James, O. (2007) *Affluenza*, London: Vermilion.

—— (2008) *The selfish capitalist*, London: Vermilion.

Kelly, G. A. (1955) *The psychology of personal constructs*, New York: Norton.

Kendell, R. E. and Zealley, A. K. (eds) (1993) *Companion to psychiatric studies*, 5th edition, Edinburgh: Churchill Livingstone.

Kennard, D. (1999) *An introduction to therapeutic communities*, London: Jessica Kingsley.

Kerr, I. B. (1999) 'Cognitive-analytic therapy for borderline personality disorder in the context of a community mental health team: individual and organizational psychodynamic implications', *British Journal of Psychotherapy* 15: 425–38.

—— (2000) 'Vygotsky, activity theory and the therapeutic community', *Therapeutic Communities* 21: 151–64.

Kerr, I. B., Dent-Brown, K. and Parry, G. D. (2007) 'Psychotherapy and mental health teams', *International Review of Psychiatry* 19: 63–80.

Kerr. I. B. and Leighton, T. (2008) 'Dual challenge: a cognitive analytic therapy approach to substance abuse', *Health Care Counselling and Psychotherapy Journal* 8: 3–7.

Kerr, I. B. and Ryle, A. (2005) 'Cognitive analytic therapy', in S. Bloch (ed.) *Introduction to the psychotherapies*, Oxford: Oxford University Press.

Kirmeyer, L. J. (1989) 'Cultural variations in the response to psychiatric disorder and mental distress', *Social Science and Medicine* 29: 327–9.

—— (2005) 'Culture, context and experience in psychiatric diagnosis', *Psychopathology* 38: 192–6.

Leahy, R. L. (2001) *Overcoming resistance in cognitive therapy*, New York: Guilford Press.

Leiman, M. (1992) 'The concept of sign in the work of Vygotsky, Winnicott and Bakhtin: further integration of object relations theory and activity theory', *British Journal of Medical Psychology* 65: 209–21.

—— (2004) 'Dialogical sequence analysis', in H. Hermans and G. Dimaggio (eds) *The dialogical self in psychotherapy*, Hove: Brunner-Routledge.

Marcuse, H. (1964) *One dimensional man*, London: Routledge.

Marmot, M. and Wilkinson, R. (2006) *Social determinants of health*, 2nd edition, Oxford: Oxford University Press.

McLaren, N. (1998) 'A critical review of the biopsychosocial model', *Australian and New Zealand Journal of Psychiatry* 32: 86–92.

Meares, R. (1998) 'The self in conversation: on narratives, chronicles and scripts', *Psychoanalytic Dialogues* 8: 875–91.

Millon, T. (1993) 'The borderline personality: a psychosocial epidemic', in J. Paris (ed.) *Borderline personality disorder: etiology and treatment*, Washington, DC: American Psychiatric Press.

Mitchell, S. A. (2000) *Relationality: from attachment to intersubjectivity*, Hillsdale, NJ: The Analytic Press.

Moos, R. H. (2008) 'Active ingredients of substance use-focused self-help groups', *Addiction* 103: 387–96.

Orford, J. (2008) 'Asking the right questions in the right way: the need for a shift in research on psychological treatments for addiction', *Addiction* 103: 875–85.

Parker, I. (ed.) (1998) *Social constructionism: discourse and reality*, London: Sage.

Putnam, R. (2000) *Bowling alone: the collapse and revival of American community*, New York: Touchstone.

Read, J., Van Os, J., Morrison, A. and Ross, C. A. (2005) 'Childhood trauma, psychosis and schizophrenia. A literature review with theoretical and clinical implications', *Acta Psychiatrica Scandinavica* 112: 330–50.

Reddy, V. (2008) *How infants know minds*, Cambridge, MA: Harvard University Press.

Rizzolatti, G. and Craighero, L. (2004) 'The mirror neuron system', *Annual Review of Neuroscience* 27: 169–92.

Rogoff, B. (2003) *The cultural nature of human development*, Oxford: OUP.

Rutter, M. (2000) 'Psychosocial influences: critiques, findings and research needs', *Development and Psychopathology* 12: 375–405.

Ryle, A. and Kerr, I. B. (2002) *Introducing cognitive analytic therapy: principles and practice*, Chichester, NY: John Wiley and Sons.

Schweder, R. A. and Bourne, E. J. (1982) 'Does the concept of the person vary cross-culturally?', in A. J. Marsella and G. M. White (eds) *Cultural conceptions of mental health and therapy*, Dordrecht: Reidel.

Shotter, J. and Gergen, K. J. (eds) (1989) *Texts of identity*, London: Sage.

Stacey, R. (2003) *Complexity and group processes: a radically social understanding of individuals*, Hove: Brunner Routledge.

Stern, D. N. (2000) *The interpersonal world of the infant: a view from psychoanalysis and developmental psychology*, 2nd edition, New York: Basic Books.

Stevens, A. and Price, J. (1996) *Evolutionary psychiatry, a new beginning*, London: Routledge.

Stiles, W. (1997) 'Signs and voices: joining a conversation in progress', *British Journal of Medical Psychotherapy* 70: 169–76.

Summerfield, D. (2001) 'The invention of post-traumatic stress disorder and the social usefulness of a psychiatric category', *British Medical Journal* 322: 95–8.

—— (2004) 'Cross cultural perspectives on the medicalization of human suffering', in G. Rosen (ed.) *PTSD – issues and controversies*, Chichester: John Wiley.

Thomas, P. and Bracken, P. (2004) 'Critical psychiatry in practice', *Advances in Psychiatric Treatment* 10: 361–70.

Thompson, A., Donnison, J., Warnock-Parkes, E., Turpin, G., Turner, J. and Kerr, I. B. (2008) 'Multidisciplinary community mental health team's experience of a skills level training course in cognitive analytic therapy', *International Journal of Mental Health Nursing* 17: 131–7.

Trevarthen, C. and Aitken K. J. (2001) 'Infant intersubjectivity: research, theory and clinical applications', *Journal of Child Psychology and Psychiatry* 42: 3–48.

Vygotsky, L. S. (1978) *Mind in society. The development of higher psychological processes*, Cambridge, MA: Harvard University Press.

Warner, R. (1994) *Recovery from schizophrenia: psychiatry and political economy*, 2nd edition, London: Routledge.

Weich, S. and Lewis, G. (1998) 'Poverty, unemployment and the common mental disorders. A population based study', *British Medical Journal* 317: 115–19.

Whitley, R. and Mackenzie, K. (2005) 'Social capital and psychiatry: review of the literature', *Harvard Review of Psychiatry* 13: 71–84.

Wilkinson, R. G. (2005) *The impact of inequality: how to make sick societies healthier*, London and New York: Routledge.

Wilkinson, R. and Pickett, K. (2009) *The spirit level. Why more equal societies almost always do better*, London: Penguin Books.

Wilson, E. O. (1998) *Consilience. The unity of knowledge*, London: Abacus.

Part IV

Questioning the orthodoxies of collaboration

Chapter 10

Transforming social work identities

Towards a European model?

Mark Smith

Introduction

In this chapter I chart the decline of social work in Scotland from its optimistic beginnings in the Social Work (Scotland) Act (1968) to the present where it is described as a 'profession lacking in confidence in its own skills and unclear about its distinctive contribution' (SE 2006a: 14). I focus on social work with children and families addressing the retreat from a welfare discourse to one of neoliberal consumerism – a shift which is made manifest in fragmented discourses around children and how best to respond to their needs and which has also impacted on social workers' professional identities. Declining trust in welfare professionals, spawning rafts of regulation and scrutiny has, I suggest, contributed to the air of pessimism that permeates state social work across the UK polities. Against this backdrop, I discuss the possibilities offered by European models of social pedagogy as providing an alternative paradigm for work with children and families. Ideas at the core of such European models, I argue, resonate with Scottish welfare traditions.

Kilbrandon

Many of the principles and provisions of the Social Work (Scotland) Act (1968), Scottish social work's foundational legislation, can be traced back to the *Kilbrandon Report* (1964). Lord Kilbrandon was commissioned by John Maclay, then Secretary of State for Scotland, 'to consider the provisions of the law of Scotland relating to the treatment of juvenile delinquents and juveniles in need of care or protection or beyond parental control' (Kilbrandon 1964: vii). The Kilbrandon committee concluded that similarities in the underlying situation of juvenile offenders and children in need of care and protection 'far outweigh the differences' and that 'the true distinguishing factor . . . is their need for special measures of education and training, the normal up-bringing processes having, for whatever reason, fallen short' (ibid.: 9).

Kilbrandon's conception of education extended beyond teaching, but was 'education in its widest sense', social education, of 'the whole child', to support the process of 'upbringing' (ibid.: 8). It was 'to include all children whose educational requirements are not met by the normal educational processes of the home or school' (ibid.: 9). Social work thus drew, from its inception, on an extant educational tradition (Smith and Whyte 2008). Education was thus seen as happening at home as well as at school. The remedy for a failure in 'upbringing', was 'social education', additional measures of education for the child, and where appropriate for the parents, in order to strengthen 'those natural influences for good which will assist the child's development into a mature and useful member of society' (Kilbrandon 1964: 9). Needs rather than deeds were to be the touchstone for intervention, and it was this principle that underpinned the introduction, in 1971, of children's hearings as the community response to children deemed to have offended or to be in need of care and protection. The hearings system reflected a contextual morality, which conceived that behaviours could only be understood in the context of the social circumstances from which they arose (Smith and Whyte 2008). The matching field organization to support this social education function was designated the Social Education Department, which was to be located in local authorities under the Director of Education and staffed by social workers (Kilbrandon 1964). Thus, social work with children and families was conceived as broadly educational and was to take place within a universal education system.

Social work and the community

While there can be a tendency nowadays to portray Kilbrandon's ideas as radical, they evince, more than anything perhaps, a somewhat patrician common sense. The 1960s, however, marked the high point of welfare consensus, reflecting a belief that the welfare state could eradicate what Beveridge had identified as the five scourges of want, disease, squalor, ignorance and idleness (UK Parliament 1942). A powerful social work lobby with visions of 'cradle to grave' welfare services emerged from this heady mix. Social work as a profession was viewed as a positive and radical force for social change (Brodie, Nottingham and Plunkett 2008). In this climate Kilbrandon's concept of social education was considered too limiting. The Association of Child Care Officers (ACCO) took the view that 'social work goes much beyond the boundaries of social education and cannot be embraced by it even considered in its widest sense' (cited in Hiddleston 2006: n.p.). ACCO argued that: 'Measures more radical, more logical than proposed by the committee, *viz.* all the social services should be concentrated in one department' (ibid.). This more radical view held sway and was incorporated into the UK Parliament White Paper, *Social Work and the Community* (1966), (subsequently enshrined in the Social Work (Scotland) Act (1968), enacted in 1971), which adopted some of Kilbrandon's ideas, but located them within generic social work departments.

The Social Work (Scotland) Act (1968)

The 1968 Act placed a broad duty on local authorities to promote social welfare. The enactment of this Act represents the high point in Scottish social work, which, especially following the inception of regional authorities in 1975, enjoyed a place at the top table in the local authority hierarchy (Brodie *et al.* 2008). The optimism which this lent to the profession supported a range of responses and developments. A collective dimension became apparent in practice in the growth of community social work, especially in the West of Scotland. In child care, a group of psychologists attached to 'List D Schools' (the successors to approved schools, residential institutions for young offenders, following the 1968 Act) drew on the spirit of Kilbrandon and on the work of the Scottish Institute of Human Relations to develop distinctively Scottish approaches to working with children and families that were developmentally based; while the newly established children's hearings system, under the guidance of some impressive founding Reporters to the Children's Panel, brought a genuinely 'whole child' perspective to deliberations about how best to deal with children in trouble or in need of care. However, a radical element, linking a structural analysis of clients' problems to an ethical imperative to act to address these problems, raised questions about the profession's role as operating both in and against the state (Lavalette and Ferguson 2007).

Such developments in social work were but one strand in a public sector tradition in Scotland which drew together different government departments in pursuit of a common good. As Paterson says,

> Links among 'physical, mental and emotional well-being' also underpinned the child-centred ideas that grew to dominate educational policy by the 1960s, reaching their apogee in the relatively successful and popular Scottish system of comprehensive secondary schools – a policy entirely based on the premise that educational success and failure cannot be understood only in educational terms, but must be related to the social and economic circumstances faced by children. From that same time, too, we have the internationally respected Scottish system of community education, linking education, youth work and community development in an attempt to regenerate whole communities, enabling them to take responsibility for their own lives.
>
> (Paterson 2000: n.p.)

However, other strands were critical in the development of social work. The new profession was regulated at a UK-wide level by the Central Council for Education and Training in Social Work (CCETSW) and, unlike education, this body lacked a discrete identity in Scotland. Social work in the UK had been heavily influenced by the American psychosocial tradition (Higham 2001) and practice developed, primarily, along casework models with responses to social problems taking the form of individual or family counselling interventions. The relationship of social work with the educational establishment in Scotland was also ambivalent from the outset. List D schools for instance were not brought under social work control and indeed strongly resisted this move, regarding social work as almost parvenu in its understanding of how best to work with 'delinquent children', and clinging to the ideal of support for such children being best undertaken within a universal education service. And, of course, the creation of a new social work profession did indeed have the effect of removing children who offended or were in need of care from the scope of such a universal education service. Thus, children came to be engaged with by social workers on the basis of their presenting difficulties rather than such difficulties being regarded as indicative of a need for additional measures of social education.

The new Right

The election of a Conservative government in 1979, led by Margaret Thatcher, saw the very precepts of social work threatened by the growth of neoliberal ideas and a concomitant retreat from welfare principles. At one level this is apparent in the increasing marketization of social work at that time. The centrality of the market was expressed too in the doctrine of managerialism, 'a set of beliefs and practices at the core of which burns the seldom tested assumption that better management will prove an effective solvent for a wide range of economic and social ills' (Pollitt 1990: 1). Managerial principles can be seductive, appealing to a common-sense view of the world, professing a 'globalising and imperialistic logic that proclaims itself as the universally applicable solution to the problems of efficiency, incompetence and chaos in the old ways of providing public services' (Clarke 1998: 174). And in many respects social work was seduced.

The seduction was made possible as a result of what Clarke and Newman (1997) describe as the ability of the proponents of neoliberalism to present their own proposals as progressive. Aspiring to provide choice, meet consumer demand and empower the individual assumed a freshness when set against the bureaucracy and inefficiency ascribed to the welfare system. At a practical level the quest for a punchier, more focused social work practice was manifest in a shift away from generic social work to services based around particular client groupings. Thus, the children and families focus, which had been deemed inadequate and limiting in the post-Kilbrandon debates, now became the norm.

The modernizing agenda

The New Labour government, which came to power in 1997, led by Tony Blair, introduced a different language to the public services, ostensibly moving away from reductionist considerations of cost to take into account broader criteria around value. In Scotland, the modernizing agenda is set out in the White Paper, *Aiming for Excellence* (SO 1999), which proposed that social work can make a key contribution to social inclusion. The social work task was deemed to be complex, requiring a 'competent, confident workforce' (ibid.: para. 1.3), a phrase that featured heavily in rationalizations for subsequent workforce regulation. Orthodoxies around 'partnership' and 'joined-up working' also began to emerge. The language in the White Paper of responsiveness, delivery, reliability and continuous improvement points to the dominant consumerist thread within New Labour's approach to the public services. An obvious illustration of this is the re-branding of clients as consumers, customers or service users.

Consumerist and inclusion discourses, however, are not self-evidently progressive. Levitas (1998) identifies how notions of social inclusion shift the policy focus away from addressing poverty and inequality towards raising individual opportunities and emphasizing individual responsibilities. There is, moreover, a strong moralizing dimension to the emphasis on responsibility, and those who verge outwith the moral centre ground are subject to a range of authoritarian responses (Butler and Drakeford

2001). Indeed those who fail to measure up to the consumerist precepts of the neoliberal state, Bauman's (1998) 'flawed consumers', are positioned within an underclass, of antisocial youth, young offenders or abusive parents. Where Kilbrandon had emphasized a contextual morality, New Labour identified the poor as authors of their own misfortune, expected to take responsibility for it.

For all its promise of modernized, and by implication more efficient and streamlined, ways of delivering public services, New Labour across the UK in fact presided over a massive increase in regulatory regimes in social care (Humphrey 2003), trends reflected in the post-devolution settlement in Scotland after 1999 but especially during Jack McConnell's period as First Minister of Scotland from 2001 until 2007. A focus on information gathering and target setting entrenched bureaucratic ways of working, betraying a political culture of encroaching, insidious control. This focus on control highlights implications for professional identity, a point I return to later. The retreat from a welfare discourse, rather than bringing about more effective and efficient services, has actually led to their increasing fragmentation (Orme 2001). It has also brought about the fragmentation of Kilbrandon's redefining conception of the 'whole' child.

Fragmenting the child

Ferguson (2007) identifies a tendency of governments to co-opt what he calls persuasive words or discourses in support of political ends. Services for children and families have, over the past 30 years, shifted from a conceptual underpinning stressing the 'whole child' to being identified with the warmly persuasive, yet ultimately partial and atomizing, discourses of rights and protection. On the surface, few might be against according children appropriate rights or protection. However, such discourses are problematic when they become the primary lenses through which to view children within a neoliberal political agenda. While Jackson (2004) highlights an emphasis in the *Kilbrandon Report* and the children's panel hearings system on children's social and cultural rights, in a neoliberalist agenda the focus is narrowed to an individualistic and legalistic conception of rights. The Children (Scotland) Act (1995), which updated the Social Work (Scotland) Act (1968) in relation to children and families, marks a shift from a welfare base towards 'a justice-oriented approach in child-care decision-making where legal principles are uppermost' (McGhee and Waterhouse 1998: 49). In the current moment, the children's hearings system model of practice in Scotland is under threat, on the one hand from an increasingly correctional impulse imported from England and the US, but on the other, from a rights lobby concerned that the welfare focus of the system does not adequately safeguard children's legal rights. 'Rights', within such a paradigm reflect an 'increasing recourse to law as a means of mediating relationships . . . premised on particular values and a particular understanding of the subject as a rational, autonomous individual' (Dahlberg and Moss 2005: 30). Viewed as such, 'rights' are arguably inimical to wider concerns based around notions of care or relationship. Children, within a neoliberal rights discourse, are also, according to Goldson (2002), subject to inappropriate 'adulterising' and 'responsibilising'. Thus, it may be argued, Kilbrandon's contextual morality is sidelined as increasing numbers of children are subject to a widening array of correctional interventions, where the only rights accorded them are those of due process.

Any progressive potential that might be ascribed to an agenda of children's rights has been hijacked as a result of rights being considered alongside the far less emancipatory discourse of protection, which currently occupies a pre-eminent position in social work. Child protection has crowded out welfare as the basis of engagement with children and families. It has also spawned its own complex and defensive bureaucracy, contributing substantially to the process-driven nature of contemporary social work (Lonne *et al.* 2009). At a wider level, discourses of protection chime with a misanthropic Zeitgeist, regarding which Tronto cautions:

> protection involves a very different conception of the relationship between an individual or group, and others than does care. Caring seems to involve taking the concerns and needs of the other as the basis for action. Protection presumes bad intentions and harm.
>
> (Tronto 1993: 104–5)

A stark example of the tendency of a protectionist discourse to proceed from a presumption of bad intent and harm is the automatic involvement of the police in child protection cases. The result of this is that problems that are almost invariably social in origin become reclassified as criminal or at least potentially so. Old-fashioned notions of poverty and disadvantage are marginalized (McGhee and Waterhouse 2007) in the new agenda of protection. Moreover, the involvement of the police in child protection is rarely as an equal partner. Garrett (2004) notes that the police now perceive themselves to be the 'lead agency' in child protection, and that social workers go along with this, to the extent of adopting police language and attitudes. And it is not just child protection that has witnessed the incursion of the police into erstwhile social work domains. The whole area of youth justice has been hived off from mainstream social work and increasingly abrogated to specialized youth justice teams and police Youth Action Teams. That problems, whether of care and protection or of juvenile delinquency, which are predominantly social in nature and ought to elicit a social or socio-educational response become conceptualized and responded to within a justice model has consequences for the type of relationships social workers establish with families and youth. These become characterized by acrimony and a lack of trust. Social work intervention has in many cases become part of the problem rather than the solution for families.

Responding to social needs as these are framed within legal and criminal discourses reflects unease with messiness and ambiguity and instead indicates a desire for certainty. Legal discourses can appear to offer more in this regard than social work. Ferguson (2004: 202), drawing on Bauman, notes that 'The paradox of child protection in liquid modernity is that its "liquidity" fully emerges at a time when organizationally it has never appeared more solid in terms of its bureaucracy.' The problem with attempts to make child protection more solid through ever more procedural guidance is that the territory on which social workers operate is 'liquid', 'ambivalence and uncertainty are its daily bread and cannot be stamped out without destroying the moral substance of responsibility' (Bauman 2000: 10). The quest to reduce complexity and ambiguity, to remove the messy bits from social work, threatens its very essence. Specifically, social work has lost the 'social' from its role. It has become co-opted to neoliberal, legalistic, individualizing and blaming ways of working. And when social work is seen as other than 'social', human qualities are lost to the extent that workers often lack basic relational and communication skills (Forrester *et al.* 2008). Motivation and moral purpose are also affected. Bauman (2000: 9) argues that when the essential human and moral aspects of care are obscured behind ever more rules and regulations 'the daily practice of social work (is made) ever more distant from its original ethical impulse'. It becomes a technical/rational task rather than a relational and moral one.

Regulating the professional

A predominant focus on child protection has acted to rein in social workers. It has established 'regimes of truth' (Foucault 1980) with regard to how they are allowed to think about or engage with children (Piper and Stronach 2008), thus defining and constraining their practice. From a teaching perspective, and one perhaps even more true of social work,

> Child Protection policies, both in their form and content, act as regulatory frameworks, which constrain and proscribe teachers' practices and . . . emphasize a 'safe' and 'risk averse' form of practice. They can also be seen as technologies of performance because they presuppose a culture of mistrust in professions.
>
> (Sachs and Mellor 2005: 149)

Social work is now regulated administratively as well as discursively. Over the years social work has advanced claims for professional status similar to that enjoyed by more established occupations by arguing for its own professional body, an aim achieved through the Regulation of Care Act (2001). Arguably social work has been short-changed. Unlike professions such as medicine and law, social work's professional body is a creature of government and positions social workers similarly so. The function of the regulation of care legislation is to monitor and control the behaviour of social workers through codes of professional conduct and fitness to practise directives. The legislation governing practice is predicated on wider meta-narratives that speak of a lack of trust in professionals and assumptions that practitioners need external surveillance to ensure that they practise safely (McLaughlin 2007).

The regulation of social work can only be understood within this broader climate of professional evaluation and surveillance, whereby the state assumes ever more control of professionals through strategies of information collection and management. Social workers have become, unequivocally, agents of the state. Indeed, Sam Galbraith, minister in the first Scottish Executive, explicitly dispelled any pretensions social workers might have harboured that they were engaged in a political activity when he stated:

> Social work services are not about redressing the major injustices in our world. Their remit is not to battle with the major forces of social exclusion. It is to promote social inclusion for each individual within their circumstances.
>
> (Galbraith, quoted in Lavalette and Ferguson 2007: 25)

The de-politicization (or arguably the re-politicization) of social work in the service of a neoliberal agenda is further advanced by developments in social work education, which has since the early 1990s become routinized, constrained within a reductionist competency framework which has seen the social scientific base of the profession subsumed within a technical/rational, managerial rubric. The result of this persistent erosion of moral purpose and petty proceduralism is the air of pessimism that pervades contemporary social work identified in *Changing Lives: 21st Century Social Work Review* (SE 2006a), discussed later.

Accommodating the new order

Cree and Davis (2007) suggest that social workers are still motivated to make a difference in the lives of those they work with. Many local authority social workers, however, have given up thinking they can do so. The creative tension that previously derived from the profession's ambiguous relationship with the state has been neutered. This has its cost. The result is a profession at odds with its espoused values. The Code of Ethics of the International Federation of Social Workers states that social workers have a responsibility to promote social justice, to challenge unjust policies and practices, to challenge social conditions that contribute to social exclusion, stigmatization or subjugation, and to work towards an inclusive society (IFSW Code of Ethics 4.2, undated). Social workers' current political and indeed professional subjugation precludes them from doing so. Bourdieu (1999) identifies the consequences of this state of affairs for social workers and teachers as a 'social suffering', where the gulf between the reality of their occupations and their professional aspirations becomes a source of acute personal discomfort; a position articulated by Nottingham (2007: 471), who says, 'Their ability to provide even the minimum service compatible with their sense of professional duty [has been] undermined by successive external impositions.' But they adapt. C. Wright Mills (1959: 168) outlines how this is achieved in situations that may be dissonant with professionals' worthier aspirations: they 'carry out [a] series of apparently rational actions without any ideas of the ends they serve, and there is increasing suspicion that those at the top as well . . . only pretend they know'. The result of this is that social work continues as an occupation but would struggle to lay claim to any wider liberal or emancipatory purpose.

Changing Lives

In June 2004, Scottish ministers in the previous Labour administration initiated a 'fundamental review of social work'. This was likened to Kilbrandon in scope, a once-in-a-generation opportunity to set the direction for the profession. The review resulted in the publication, *Changing Lives* (SE 2006a), which describes many of the problems facing social work. The review identifies a profession lacking in confidence and uncertain about its role, one that is process dominated and where negative publicity around 'failures' has led to risk-averse and blame cultures. The profession, it claims, has lost touch with some of its core purpose. The report calls for trans-formational change.

Changing Lives pushes the 'joined-up' agenda. Within this, the social work role is positioned as supporting more universal services, particularly in relation to pre-ventative rather than crisis-driven agendas.

> What is needed is a joined up approach to prevention, in which social work services better support universal services to pick up and respond to the early signs of problems as well as tackling complex problems of some individuals and communities.
>
> (SE 2006a: 42)

Elsewhere it claimed that 'Social workers never work in isolation and are always part of multi-disciplinary approaches' (ibid.: 30). Thus, social work might be thought of as providing the 'linking social capital', bringing together individuals with agencies and services they might otherwise find difficulty in accessing (cf. Catts and Ozga 2005). At the same time, however, McGhee and Waterhouse identify policy effects that appear

> to lock social work out of early intervention and prevention and to align child and family-oriented social work with those cases that have crossed over a borderline where balancing care and control and the use of involuntary measures is to the fore – the 'hard cases'.
>
> (McGhee and Waterhouse 2010: np)

Changing Lives (SE 2006a) called for a rolling back of managerial 'red tape' in order to encourage the development of autonomous accountable professionals. Leadership was couched in a language of governance set up to support devolved responsibility, in contrast to previous dominant command-and-control cultures. Of course, such ideas of devolved governance are not necessarily benign and perhaps too readily may conflate with those of surveillance. There are contradictions, too, in the call for 'autonomous professionalism' which implies scope for the application of professional judgements, while the subsequent assertion that social workers 'must always work within the rules, regulations and priorities of their employers and practise in line with the standards and codes of practice of their regulatory bodies' (ibid.: 51) draws them firmly back into line.

One aspect of the report that appealed to social workers was its assertion of the importance of what it terms 'therapeutic relationships' which, within a managerial culture, had been marginalized and subsumed within case management ways of working. The review concluded that the quality of the therapeutic relationship between social workers and individuals or families was critical (ibid.: 64).

Changing Lives further proposed a new para-professional role to undertake more routine tasks, thereby freeing up social workers to undertake key aspects of their job as outlined above. In many respects the para-professional role envisaged for social work mirrors developments in other professions, such as the law, teaching and health. The proposal might presage a situation where most direct work with clients is actually undertaken by para-professionals, leaving diminishing numbers of professionally qualified social workers to undertake what are essentially 'hard end' child protection cases rather than having a role in more preventative family support. In such a scenario para-professionals become the primary direct workers with clients.

The location of *Changing Lives* within a rubric of neoliberalism is evident in the explicit shift from *welfare* to *well-being* that it advocates. While welfare speaks of a wider social purpose, well-being, as identified in the review, focuses on the individual. Services are to be individualized through the 'personalization' agenda, increasingly a key driver in the shaping of all public services. Ferguson (2007), for example, notes that the concept of personalization has attained a place at the heart of social work policy and thinking. Despite its rise to prominence, what constitutes personalization remains unclear. According to a government discussion paper, 'Personalisation can mean a number of things to different people' (SG 2007: 1). What may be said of the personalization agenda is that it further continues the trend towards individualizing social problems and responses. Thus, *Changing Lives* refers to social workers 'helping people to become self-reliant once more' (SE 2006a: 17). The failure of the review to challenge political orthodoxies is further evidenced in its acceptance that: 'Political priorities will continue to be driven by fear of crime and anti-social behaviour' (ibid.: 21), with the concomitant that more and more young people and family members will be drawn into the criminal justice system.

So while *Changing Lives* might have been compared to *Kilbrandon* it reflects none of the latter's optimism. *Kilbrandon* was a child of its time and so too is *Changing Lives*, but it is rooted in the individualism, fragmentation, anxiety and ultimately the misanthropy of late modernity.

The working together agenda

Changing Lives identified the need for social workers to operate alongside other professionals, serving to reinforce existing orthodoxies. Menter notes that the former Scottish Executive had stated as early as 2001 that 'children's services – encompassing education, child welfare, social work, health, leisure and recreation services for children from birth to 18 years – should consider themselves as a single unitary system' (Menter 2009: 60). Administratively, children and families social work services are increasingly merged with the education service. However, the potential for a lack of shared conceptual understanding of children, childhood or families to exist among professionals working in different areas calls into question the assumption that such joint working will bring about more effective services. While integration may be happening at a policy level it is scarcely impacting on teachers' practice (see, for example, Menter 2009). The same might safely be said of inter/professional policy exhortations to social workers and other professionals working with children. So long as changes take place only at policy and organizational levels they will fail to bring about the integrated service to children and families intended by successive governments. Teachers will continue to teach and social workers will continue to process children and families through an increasingly procedural and blaming child protection system.

Christie and Menmuir (2005) question whether the integrated services agenda might be advanced by the adoption of common professional standards. Menter (2009), however, suggests that recourse to 'standards' may reinforce the increasing technical rationality of public services. A further problem with standards is that they tend to be curtailed by the limits of our thinking in respect of children and childhood, and this currently struggles to move beyond discourses of rights or protection. To address the needs of the whole child requires a shift in that thinking. Services for children and families need to be thought of within an alternative paradigm. Such a conceptual shift might take us in the direction of social education or social pedagogy.

The possibilities of social pedagogy

Social pedagogy is the discipline underpinning direct work with children and families across much of Europe, its roots stretching back to the 19th century. The aim of Johann Heinrich Pestalozzi, a founding pedagogue, was to educate the whole child, embracing three elements – hands, heart and head; principles that remain central to current notions of social pedagogy (Petrie 2004). Social pedagogues were 'educators of the poor' working in special schools but also in poor rural areas. Education was seen as central to social development and the creation of community. Smith and Whyte (2008: 19) note that Diesterweg, a Prussian educator, argued that social pedagogy should be expressed in 'educational action by which one aims to help the poor in society'. Thus, social pedagogy aims to promote social welfare through broadly based socio-educational strategies, providing a framework for the consideration of the individual in society and thus offering a counterpoint to the individually atomizing tendencies of neoliberalism. In that sense it has the potential to put the 'social' back into social work.

Social pedagogical ideas increasingly merit a mention in discussion of integrated service provision. The *Getting it Right for Every Child* policy document (SE 2006b) introduces a national agenda in Scotland for all professionals working with children, identifying the need for multi-systemic approaches to meet the range of needs. While within this context the concept of social pedagogy potentially offers a useful way forward, concerns might arise if that approach were seen solely as a solution to the problems of inter/professional working rather than being grounded in any deeper understanding of the concept of social pedagogy and its concern to educate all elements of the child.

Social work as social education

At a time when the future of social work is uncertain, ideas of social pedagogy or social education may offer possibilities for its future direction. The literature review on the role of the social worker, undertaken for *Changing Lives* (Asquith, Clark and Waterhouse 2005: 24), argues that social pedagogy emphasizes 'working directly with people much as promised by the core values of social work', values that are acknowledged as having been diminished in the profession's recent history.

Adopting ideas of social pedagogy would require that social work be thought of as an essentially educational undertaking. Cree makes this point, arguing:

> When we stop seeing social work as a narrow, municipally based, bureaucratic activity, we start to see that it is, at its deepest level, a form of education . . . what might be called 'social education' – it has been about getting alongside people in a process of change, about bringing about change, within individuals and communities.
>
> (Cree 2008: np)

Locating social work within a broadly educational framework resonates with Scottish traditions of education and social welfare. There are persistent points of departure between Scottish approaches and dominant Anglo-American models. There are perhaps two defining differences, which derive from different attitudes towards education. In contrast to Anglo-American models, in Scotland education has been viewed as a collective rather than an individual enterprise, 'having a key role in tackling a range of social problems and in promoting cohesion in a more diverse society' (Bloomer 2008: 32). The other defining difference relates to a philosophical predisposition in Scotland towards what might be viewed as a contextual morality, which takes into account social circumstances in judging behaviours rather than reliance on more abstract and universalist principles (Smith and Whyte 2008).

Both these dimensions are evident in the proposals for social education departments put forward in the *Kilbrandon Report* (1964). They are also reflected in mainstream European approaches to working with children and families. Asquith *et al.* suggest that:

> There are grounds to believe that what [Kilbrandon] intended was not an 'education' department in the traditional sense but rather a department based on principles much akin to those of social pedagogy. The social education department proposed by Kilbrandon may well have had its roots more in the notion of allowing an individual to realise his/her potential in society, much as with the role of the 'educateur' in France.
>
> (Asquith *et al.* 2005: 23)

The return of social work practice to the principles contained within the Kilbrandon report acknowledges the fundamental soundness of proposals that were never fully realized within social work. Reclaiming Kilbrandon's ideas and articulating the consonance between these and ideas of social pedagogy might allow social work to reinvigorate some of its original aspirations. Social pedagogy is not necessarily a direct alternative to social work but potentially may offer 'a mirror in which the social work tradition can become aware of its own rich but also contested diversity that already contains many of the same elements as the social pedagogy tradition' (Lorenz 2008: 641).

The time is perhaps apposite for a shift in the direction of social pedagogy. The Scottish Nationalist Party (SNP) government elected in Scotland in 2007 and re-elected for a second term in 2011, professes itself to be a social democratic party with 'radical social ambitions' (Salmond 2007), determined to consider distinctively Scottish approaches to service provision and delivery. In some policy areas the Scottish government looks to Nordic countries with well-established social welfare systems based around social pedagogy. William Roe (2008) who chaired the *Changing Lives* report suggests that the current Scottish government is disposed to explore methods for building common values and language between professionals. He goes on to say that he would have liked *Changing Lives* to recommend a professional

> equipped to work with children and families across all disciplines that make up the children's service sector. There remain a lot of professional barriers between distinct disciplines in Scotland and the pedagogue model . . . could, over time, help to break these down.
>
> (Roe 2008: 37)

The children's charity, Children in Scotland (2008), explicitly advocates the adoption of a 'Scottish Pedagogue' model of the professional working with children. However, there remains resistance to this, much of it converging around how well understood the term 'social pedagogue' might be in Scotland. Yet in failing to call it by name the impact of adopting social pedagogic ideas is likely to be lessened.

Unifying concepts: 'upbringing' and '*Bildung*'

An attraction of social pedagogy is that its central ideas, those of 'upbringing', and '*Bildung*' – a concept which encompasses notions of learning, socialization and personal development – provide unifying concepts within which to locate services for children and families. In Germany, '*Erzieher*', the term for a pedagogue, translates to 'upbringer', resonating with Kilbrandon's identification of the centrality of 'upbringing' in all work with children and families. Similarly, the German term, '*Bildung*', while not amenable to direct translation, may offer a window to Kilbrandon's idea of 'education in its widest sense', incorporating, but at the same time transcending, traditional teaching and learning also to include a sense of character and the moral formation of children as full members of society.

Ideas of upbringing and '*Bildung*' go beyond more limited discourses of rights or protection to encompass ideas regarding what more may be required for children to develop into healthy and 'competent' adults. This broader view of education, at a policy level, is perhaps evident in *Curriculum for Excellence* (SE 2004) which states its central purpose as enabling all children to become: successful learners, confident individuals, effective contributors and responsible citizens.

Conclusion

Social work, conceived as a profession at the height of modernist optimism, has fallen prey to postmodern fragmentation, anxiety and pessimism. This fragmentation can be identified at a conceptual level. The 'whole child' model of social education or 'upbringing' envisaged by the *Kilbrandon Report* and evident in European social pedagogy has been crowded out by the intellectually and morally limiting discourses of rights or protection. In this chapter, I have argued that aspirations for children are best served within broadly educational approaches to practice rather than in solutions rooted in individual or family deficit or blame, which seem to be embedded within dominant Anglo-American paradigms of social welfare.

Discursive shifts from welfare towards neoliberal consumerism have also taken their toll on professional identities. While social workers may still come into the profession determined to make a difference in people's lives they are often, it seems, ground down in a petty proceduralism that dissipates this initial moral purpose. The profession is conflicted by internal tensions where daily practice is dissonant with espoused values. We have reached a stage where social work is neither 'social', nor is it working. Its predicament perhaps opens up spaces to reclaim some of its broadly educational roots, through revisiting Kilbrandon's ideas for social education or European models of social pedagogy.

References

Asquith, S., Clark, C. and Waterhouse, L. (2005) *The role of the social worker in the 21st century*, Edinburgh: Stationery Office.
Bauman, Z. (1998) *Globalisation: The human consequences*, Cambridge: Polity Press.
—— (2000) 'Am I my brother's keeper?', *European Journal of Social Work* 3(1): 5–11.
Bloomer, K. (2008) 'Modernising Scotland's teaching workforce', in *Working it out: developing the children's sector workforce*, Edinburgh: Children in Scotland.
Bourdieu, P. (1999) *The weight of the world: social suffering in contemporary society*, Polity: Cambridge.
Brodie, I., Nottingham, C. and Plunkett, S. (2008) 'A tale of two reports: social work in Scotland from Social Work and the Community (1966) to *Changing Lives* (2006)', *British Journal of Social Work* 38: 697–715.
Butler, I. and Drakeford, M. (2001) 'Which Blair project? Communitarianism, social authoritarianism and social work', *Journal of Social Work* 1: 7–24.
Catts, R. and Ozga, J. (2005) 'What is social capital and how might it be used in Scottish Schools?', *CES Briefing* 36, Edinburgh: Centre for Educational Sociology, University of Edinburgh.
Children in Scotland (2008) *Working it out: developing the children's sector workforce*, Edinburgh: Children in Scotland.
Christie, D. and Menmuir, J. (2005) 'Supporting interprofessional collaboration in Scotland through a Common Standards Framework Policy', *Futures in Education* 3: 62–74.
Clarke, J. (1998) 'Thriving on chaos? Managerialism and the welfare state', in J. Carter (ed.) *Postmodernity and the fragmentation of welfare*, London: Routledge.
Clarke, J. and Newman, J. (1997) *The managerial state: power, politics and ideology in the remaking of social welfare*, London: Sage.

Cree, V. (2008) 'Researching social work: reflections on a contested profession', Inaugural Lecture, University of Edinburgh, 29 January 2008.

Cree, V. and Davis, A. (2007) *Social work: voices from the inside*, Abingdon: Routledge.

Dahlberg, G. and Moss, P. (2005) *Ethics and politics in early childhood education*, London: Routledge/Falmer.

Ferguson, H. (2004) *Protecting children in time: child abuse, child protection and the consequences of modernity*, Basingstoke: Palgrave Macmillan.

Ferguson, I. (2007) 'Increasing user choice or privatizing risk? The antinomies of personalization', *British Journal of Social Work* 37: 387–403.

Forrester, D., Kershaw, S., Moss, H. and Hughes, L. (2008) 'Communication skills in child protection: how do social workers talk to parents?', *Child and Family Social Work* 13: 41–51.

Foucault, M. (1980) *Power/knowledge*, New York: Pantheon.

Garrett, P. M. (2004) 'Talking child protection. The police and social workers "working together"', *Journal of Social Work* 4: 77–97.

Goldson, B. (2002) 'New Labour, social justice and children: political calculation and the deserving–undeserving schism', *British Journal of Social Work* 32: 683–95.

Hiddleston, V. (2006) 'The Social Work (Scotland) Act 1968', paper presented at the Social Work History Network, Edinburgh University, November 2006.

Higham, P. (2001) 'Changing practice and an emerging social pedagogue paradigm in England: the role of the personal advisor', *Social Work in Europe* 8: 21–31.

Humphrey, J. C. (2003) 'New Labour and the regulatory reform of social care', *Critical Social Policy* 23: 5–24.

International Federation of Social Workers (undated) *Ethics in social work. Statement of principals*. Online. Available at: http://www.ifsw.org/en/f38000027.html (accessed 15 December 2008).

Jackson, P. (2004) 'Rights and representation in the Scottish Children's Hearings System', in J. McGee, M. Mellon and B. Whyte (eds) *Meeting needs, addressing deeds – working with young people who offend*, Glasgow: NCH Scotland.

Kilbrandon, Lord C. J. D. Shaw (1964) *The Kilbrandon report: children and young persons Scotland*, Edinburgh: HMSO. Reprinted 1995. Online. Available at: http://www.scotland.gov.uk/Resource/Doc/47049/0023863.pdf (accessed 14 March 2011).

Lavalette, M. and Ferguson, I. (2007) (eds) *International social work and the radical tradition*, London: Venture Press.

Levitas, R. (1998) *The inclusive society? Social exclusion and New Labour*, Basingstoke: Macmillan.

Lonne, B., Parton, N., Thomson, J. and Harries, M. (2009) *Reforming child protection*, London: Routledge.

Lorenz, W. (2008) 'Paradigms and politics: understanding methods paradigms in an historical context: the case of social pedagogy', *British Journal of Social Work* 38: 625–44.

McGhee, J. and Waterhouse, L. (1998) 'Justice and welfare: has the Children (Scotland) Act (1995) shifted the balance?', *Journal of Social Welfare and Family Law* 20: 49–63.

—— (2007) 'Care and protection in Scottish child welfare: evidence of double jeopardy?', *European Journal of Social Work* 10: 145–60.

—— (2010) 'Locked out of prevention? The identity of child and family-oriented social work in Scottish post-devolution policy', *British Journal of Social Work*, doi:10.1093/bjsw/bcq121.

McLaughlin, K. (2007) 'Regulation and risk in social work: the General Social Care Council and the Social Care Register in context', *British Journal of Social Work* 37: 1263–77.

Menter, I. (2009) 'Service integration in schools: the Scottish scene and implications for teachers', in J. Forbes and C. Watson (eds) *Service integration in schools: research and policy discourses and future prospects*, Rotterdam: Sense.

Nottingham, C. (2007) 'The rise of the insecure professionals', *International Review of Social History* 52: 445–75.

Orme, J. (2001) 'Regulation or fragmentation? Directions for social work under New Labour', *British Journal of Social Work* 31: 611–24.

Paterson, L. (2000) 'Scottish democracy and Scottish utopias: the first year of the Scottish Parliament', *Scottish Affairs* 33: 45–61. Online. Available at: http://www.scottishaffairs. org/onlinepub/sa/paterson_sa33_aut00.html (accessed 7 November 2008).

Petrie, P. (2004) '*Pedagogy – a holistic, personal approach to work with children and young people across services; European models for practice, training, education and qualification*', London: Thomas Coram Research Unit, IoE, University of London.

Piper, H. and Stronach, I. (2008) *Don't touch! The educational story of a panic*, London: Routledge.

Pollitt, C. (1990) *Managerialism and the public services: the Anglo-American experience*, Oxford: Blackwell.

Roe, W. (2008) '21st century social work', in *Working it out: developing the children's sector workforce*, Edinburgh: Children in Scotland.

Sachs, J. and Mellor, L. (2005) 'Risk anxiety, child panic and child protection: a critical examination of policies from Queensland and New South Wales', *Journal of Education Policy* 20: 131–46.

Salmond, A. (2007) Interview with Andrew Marr, 20 May 2007. Online. Available at: news. bbc.co.uk/1/hi/programmes/sunday_am/6673891.stm (accessed 18 September 2008).

Scottish Executive (SE) (2004) *A curriculum for excellence. The curriculum review group*, Edinburgh: Scottish Executive.

—— (2006a) *Changing lives. 21st century social work review*, Edinburgh: Scottish Executive.

—— (2006b) *Getting it right for every child. An implementation plan*, Edinburgh: Scottish Executive.

Scottish Government (SG) (2007) *Service development change programme. Personalisation: an agreed understanding*. Online. Available at: http://www.socialworkscotland.org.uk/ resources/private/Personalisation.pdf (accessed 15 September 2008).

Scottish Office (SO) (1999) *Aiming for excellence: modernising social work services in Scotland*, Edinburgh: The Stationery Office.

Smith, M. and Whyte, B. (2008) 'Social education and social pedagogy: reclaiming a Scottish tradition in social work', *European Journal of Social Work* 11: 15–28.

Tronto, J. (1993) *Moral boundaries: a political argument for an ethic of care*, London: Routledge.

UK Parliament (1942) *Social insurance and allied services. Report by Sir William Beveridge*, London: HMSO.

Wright Mills, C. (1959) *The sociological imagination*, New York: Oxford University Press.

Chapter 11

Emergent spaces
Looking for the civic and the civil in initial professional education

Julie Allan

Please do not shoot the pianist. He is doing his best.
> (Sign seen by Oscar Wilde in a saloon bar in Leadville, Colorado, 1883)

The only thing to do, if you want to contribute to culture, or politics, or music, or whatever, is to utilize your own persona rather than just music. The best way to do this is to diversify and become a nuisance everywhere.
> (David Bowie 1976: 338)

Introduction: the donnish decline?

The role of the academic within universities has become increasingly constrained by the 'audit culture' (Strathern 1997: 305), what they write and for whom is more closely circumscribed than ever before, and the pressure to demonstrate 'impact', whatever that may be, limits their capacity to have any real influence on communities and on their values. Halsey (1992: 258) bemoans the 'decline of the donnish domin- ion', while Furedi (2004: vii) wonders 'where have all the intellectuals gone?' The undermining of academic culture and autonomy (Paterson 2003) and the regulatory practices within universities is 'producing fear and little else' (Evans 2004: 63) and is 'killing thinking' (ibid.) and, as Lyotard (1986) notes, in a world in which success is equated with saving time, thinking itself reveals its fundamental flaw to be its capacity to waste time. Edward Said (1994: 55) argues that a further danger for the intellectual comes from the limitations and constraints of professionalism which encourage conformity rather than critique:

> The particular threat to the intellectual today, whether in the West or the non- Western world, is not the academy, nor the suburbs, not the appalling com- mercialism of journalism and publishing houses, but rather an attitude that I will call professionalism. By professionalism I mean thinking of your work as an intellectual as something you do for a living, between the hours of nine and five with one eye on the clock, and another cocked at what is considered to be proper, professional behaviour – not rocking the boat, not straying outside the accepted paradigms or limits, making yourself marketable and above all presentable, hence uncontroversial and unpolitical and 'objective'.

The civic duty which was behind the creation of universities in Scotland, other parts of Europe and the US, in what was known as 'democratic intellectualism' (Paterson 2003: 69), appears to have been lost. It might be questioned, however, whether UK and US universities have ever fostered the kind of intellectualism which has been seen in French universities, through for example the likes of Foucault, Derrida and Deleuze, or those emanating from the Frankfurt school such as Habermas and Adorno. The contemporary German theorist Sloterdijk (1988), whose book, *Critique of Cynical Realism*, was bought in vast quantities by a public tempted into philosophy, has no parallels in either the UK or the US, although writers such as Michael Apple, Terry Eagleton and Slavoj Žižek appear to have made some inroads into the public imagination through their engagement with the media. E. P. Thompson is somewhat damning of those who inhabit the UK universities:

> I have never ceased to be astounded when observing the preening and mating habits of fully grown specimens of the species *Academicus superciliosis*. The behaviour patterns of one of the true members of the species are unmistakable. He is inflated with self-esteem and perpetually self-congratulatory as to the high vocation of the university teacher; but he knows almost nothing about any other vocation, and he will lie down and let himself be walked over if anyone enters from the outer world who has money or power or even a tough line in realist talk . . . *superciliosis* is the most divisible and reliable creature in this country, being so intent upon crafty calculations of short-term advantages – this favour for his department, that a colleague who, next week, at the next committee, has promised to run a log for him, that he has never even tried to imagine the wood out of which his timber rolls. He can scurry furiously and self-importantly around in his committees, like a white mouse running in a wheel, while his master is carrying him, cage and all, to be sold at the local pet-shop.
>
> (E. P. Thompson 1970: 154)

Although Thompson's observations pertain to an earlier period, the simultaneous self-importance and willingness to be bought are sinister features of contemporary academic life. Žižek (2005: 23) offers a more recent, but equally damming, account of the:

> Prattling classes, academics and journalists with no specialist education, usually working in humanities with some vague French postmodern leanings, specialists in everything, prone to verbal radicalism, in love with paradoxical formulations that flatly contradict the obvious.

Such disenchantment with academics seems unfair and misplaced since the greater problem may be their apathy and unwillingness to face up to their civic duty. Performativity may have become a convenient justification for lassitude.

Inter/professional practice in the academy

Academics involved in initial professional education face a number of pressures. They are expected to 'deliver' people to the profession in an appropriate state and having reached an acceptable standard of expertism. As Britzman (1986) notes, the cultivation of the teacher as expert promotes individualistic development at the expense of any communitarian orientation and helps to reify both knowledge and the knower. Furthermore, the cultivation of the new professional, in teaching or in other areas, encourages an aspiration to enter what Diken and Bagge Lausten have described as 'camps' which simultaneously create belonging and displacement:

> This experience of displacement is increasingly threatened within the horizon of 'camping' today insofar as the camp bypasses the city as a space of exposure and touching. The logic of (self-)exemption tends to turn difference into indifference, while otherness is 'tolerated' but walled-off. The 'tolerance' of the camp neatly places every culture on its own turf in a mosaic bereft of interaction. In its horizon, in other words, tolerance cannot become solidarity and forced contingency cannot turn into a chosen destiny . . . The camp . . . makes it impossible to confront others and to take moral/political choices, because its logic defines the others before they are met.
>
> (Diken and Bagge Lausten 2005: 1)

Initial teacher education programmes are packed increasingly tightly to ensure each new policy imperative is covered, but there are few possibilities for removal to make space for the new additions. Furthermore, there is no incentive or opportunity to allow beginning teachers to engage with educational theory. There is no room within the curriculum for this and the material resources for teaching are theoretically light and amount to 'theory junk sculpture' (Thomas 2008: 1). The plethora of handbooks, promising such goodies as *Six Principles for Teaching English Language Learners in all Classrooms* (McIntyre *et al.* 2008), *60 Research-based Teaching Strategies that Help Special Learners Succeed* (McNary 2005) or *Commonsense Methods for Children with Special Educational Needs* (Westwood 2002), present teaching as technical matter and offer no more than simplistic sound bites about teaching. As Brantlinger (2006: 45) points out, textbooks – the 'big glossies' – function as 'authoritative purveyors of technical knowledge' (ibid.: 67) and portray idealized versions of classroom life and of children benefiting from interventions. These are presented as having a sound theoretical base, but as Thomas (2008: 1) observes, they offer beginning teachers a 'cacophony of incompatible explanations', which amount to 'a bazaar . . . in which plausible homily, mixed with large portions of psychoanalytic and psychological vocabulary, take the place of a rational consideration of children's behaviour at school'. Gregoriou notes the increasingly widespread demand for the simple, the practical and the reducible which:

> Threatens to totalize experience, to reduce language to Newspeak, to rob thinking of its childhood and pedagogy of its philosophical moment. It is the 'demand'

for reality (for unity, simplicity, communicability) and remedy: remedy for the parcelling and virtualization of culture, for the fragmentation of the life world and its derealization into idioms, *petits recits*, and language games.

(Gregoriou 2004: 233, original emphasis)

This demand for simplification is accompanied by a resistance to thinking and, as Colebrook (2006: 2) suggests, 'all around us . . . we encounter the absence of thinking, the malevolence and stupidity that go well beyond error'. Goodson (2003: 9) accuses teacher educators of having submitted to a practice ethos and 'surrendered their theoretical missions', while Hirst (1989: 272) bemoans the fact that in-service teacher education is 'now concentrating severely on the practical demands of new legislation . . . Advanced study of a systematic kind is now much reduced.' According to Greene, this has created a displacement of teacher education from both the public and teachers themselves:

> There are moments when many of us sense an odd distance between the ethos of teacher education and lived lives of the publics to whom we hope the schools can respond. There are moments when I feel a similar gap between ourselves and many of the teachers in those schools. I have some of our normatives in mind, our styles of explanations, our ways of putting things.
>
> (Greene 1991: 541)

Goodson sees collaborative work as the only way in which teacher educators can be rescued and allowed to reconnect with educational theory in ways which will make practice more meaningful.

The individualistic approach to initial professional education provides little incentive to beginning professionals to consider those in other professions. The *Standard for Full Registration* (GTCS 2006a), against which Scottish teachers are judged, includes an element of working co-operatively with other professionals and adults. However, in order to meet this particular element teachers merely have to demonstrate that they can 'create and sustain appropriate working relationships with other teachers, support staff and visiting professionals' (ibid.: 10). Such low expectations in relation to inter/professional practice, together with the scarce mention of other professionals, and even then only as generalized others, will inevitably leave the beginning teacher surmising that a lack of importance is given to this work. This othering of professionals with whom teachers are supposed to engage 'appropriately', seen in the *Standard for Full Registration*, is continued in the *Standard for Chartered Teacher* (GTCS 2006b). However, in order to gain this enhanced status, teachers are expected to exert an 'influence' on these generalized others. The influence does not appear to be a benign one. Elsewhere in the UK the intention to incorporate inter/professional collaboration within teacher education standards has been expressed (UCET 2003; Moran and Abbott 2006), but as Moran, Abbott and O'Connor (2009) observe, progress on this front has been extremely slow.

There are many enjoinders, within policies, to undertake inter/professional practice, to collaborate, or to engage in 'joined-up' working (Makareth and Turner 2002; Milne 2005). For example, the report of Her Majesty's Inspectorate of

Education (2002), *Count Us In: Achieving Inclusion in Scottish Schools*, identifies integrated service provision as essential for inclusion, while *Educating for Excellence, Choice and Opportunity* (SE 2003) calls for professionals in health, education and social work to work together in the interests of young people. There is, however, limited knowledge about how to engage in inter/professional working practices and little evidence about the impact such efforts might have on the children and families they are supposed to support. The language used in these policies – of joined-up working, the 'whole' child and initiatives being rolled out – the last of which, as Daniels (2005) suggests, conjures up notions of laying carpets and ensuring all the bumps are ironed out, privileges consensus and creates closure. Joined-up working in particular appears to be more of a cliché than a policy, ordered by government departments which are themselves disconnected and function within cells.

In spite of the absence of any clear rationale for inter/professional practice, knowledge of how to do this and evidence of impact, there appears to be a generally positive regard for it. However, academics who have taken on the task of promoting inter/professional practice may have inadvertently descended into emotivism, which Alasdair MacIntyre (1984) describes as a confusion between two kinds of reply to the question 'Why should I do . . .?' The first reply takes the form of 'Because I wish it' and is confined to the personal context of the utterance and the characteristics of the speaker. The second reply is unconditional and independent of who utters it, taking the form of 'Because it is your duty.' MacIntyre suggests that the second reply is often used to mean 'I like it and urge it on or recommend it to you' (Hernstein Smith 1992). Inter/professional practice, in this respect, is urged and pressed on people under the guise of a well argued and *moral* evaluation; and arguments, which may be fallacious, in the sense of having an error in reasoning on material, psychological or logical grounds (Fearnside and Holther 1959), are constructed to trick people into accepting inter/professional practice as a good thing. This is potentially effective:

> Here is another trick, which, as soon as it is practicable, makes all others unnecessary. Instead of working on your opponent's intellect by argument, work on his will by motive, and he, and also the audience if they have similar interests, will at once be won over by your opinion, even though you got it out of a lunatic asylum.
>
> (Schopenhauer 1896: xxxv)

Emotivism, according to MacIntyre, is a widespread phenomenon, but it leaves an overwhelming sense of confusion and of having been deceived:

> Now people still say 'It is good' and *think* they mean 'It is good', but, without knowing, they are really doing only what people used to do when they said 'I like it' or 'I want it', namely expressing their own feelings and trying to get other people to feel, do, or believe certain things. And everyone is deceived: listeners are deceived about what speakers are doing; speakers are self-deceived about what they themselves are doing; and moral philosophers are either deceived, complacent, or complicitous.
>
> (Hernstein Smith 1992: 213–14, original emphasis)

The external pressures upon academics concerned with initial professional education, together with those they create for themselves, appear to be enormous and are likely to produce both frustration and impotence. However, Bourdieu (1998: 128) maintains that it is vital that they are protected from urgent duties and that they can be allowed to 'play seriously': '*Homo scholasticus* or *Homo academicus* is someone who can play seriously because his or her state (or State) assures her the means to do so, that is, free time, outside the urgency of a practical situation.'

So how might academics regain control, rediscover their civic duty and engage in serious play? I want to suggest three possible kinds of reorientations which academics themselves might be able to effect. These concern the ontological (their own selves and others), the epistemological (knowledge) and the epiphanic (the unforeseen and inaccessible aspects of ordinary life).

An 'other' ontology

On a basic level, academics concerned with initial professional education and inter/professional practice might ask 'What *can* we do?' and, to respond to that question effectively, I am suggesting that what is required is an ontological reorientation of themselves as political individuals who must *act* and who, in order to do so, will have to realign themselves in the academic and professional world. To effect these realignments, initial professional education might be conceived of as an ethical project, using the framework offered by Foucault (1984, 1994), and in which one's own self – and one's capacity to be in relation to others – is considered part of the material on which work has to be done (Allan 2005, 2008). Maxine Greene (2008: n.p.) offers a helpful construction of the becoming nature of the self: 'I am what I am not yet.' What seems necessary is both desire for inter/professional practice and an undertaking to enact that desire on behalf of others. To return to MacIntyre's question of 'Why should I do?' the academic's answer may become a purposeful elision which avoids emotivism because the imperative is directed back towards themselves. In other words, 'Because I wish it' and 'Because it is *my* duty.'

Academics may find it difficult to act politically within their own institutions, but there are multiple ways in which they might oppose institutional practices which are restrictive (Ballard 2003; Brantlinger 2006) and encourage 'communication across a multiplicity of cultures, identities and ways of thinking' (Booth 2003: 55). Apple (2001) recommends that we face up to the dynamics of power in unromantic ways, and promotes the use of subversive tactics to challenge the hegemonic order, including tactical and counter-hegemonic alliances and heretical thought. He also suggests that while we might recapture our past to see what is possible, it is important not to romanticize dreams about the future. Corbett and Slee's (2000: 134) depiction of academics as 'cultural vigilantes' is a useful starting point and the language of enmity is appropriate as a *casus belli*, an occasion of war for which there is just cause.

Evans (2004: 309) suggests the kind of refusal of institutional power evoked by Virginia Woolf in *Three Guineas* which amounts to an 'attitude of complete indifference'. Woolf envisaged this as a war against the 'pompous and self important' (Evans 2004: 76) behaviour of males, but Evans suggests that this kind of resistance (by anyone) could be effective within universities and could lead to a different kind of politics which seeks to undermine those 'practices and processes which increasingly deform much of academic life' (ibid.: 102).

Knowing the unknowns

The lack of knowledge about what inter/professional practice entails is a serious omission which must be addressed with urgency. Furthermore, consideration needs to be given to identifying the most appropriate way to undertake the research that will obtain this knowledge (Allan 2008; Allan and Slee 2008; Gallagher 2008; Thomas 2008). Flyvbjerg (2001) suggests that judgements about the efficacy of social science research in general are based on criteria which are inappropriate and, therefore, unjust. He argues that it is compared to research within the natural science on the basis of its *episteme* (scientific knowledge) and *techne* (technical knowledge or know-how). Judgements about social science research are based on its capacity to produce explanatory and predictive theory – on its epistemic qualities. This is, he says, simply not fair, since these terms are self-defeating and whilst social science research has indeed contributed little to explanatory and predictive theory it has contributed a great deal to reflexive analysis and discussion of values and interests as *phronesis*. Flyvbjerg contends that it is social science's *phronetic* qualities, its concern for values and power, that should be evaluated and this would seem to be a more appropriate basis for undertaking research on inter/professional practice and making judgements about its quality:

> The goal is to help restore social science to its classical position as a practical, intellectual activity aimed at clarifying the problems, risks, and possibilities we face as humans and societies, and at contributing to social and political praxis.
>
> (Flyvbjerg 2001: 4)

Addressing imbalances of power between researchers and researched and ensuring that research practices are just is also vital and this requires academics to interrogate the way in which their own research positions their research subjects. New alliances with individuals, groups and organizations, and among professionals and students, which seek to flatten the division between the researcher and the researched and provide a better understanding of the potential for resistance, are necessary. There is a need to undertake analyses that uncover and do justice (in both senses) to the complexity and messiness of inter/professional practice, and the philosophers of difference – Foucault, Derrida, Deleuze and Guattari – seem to offer some considerable promise in this regard (Allan 2008, 2009). Thomas (2008: 7) has argued that instead of structured theoretical frameworks, what we need are 'simpler and looser understandings', based on a Deweyan form of investigation, while Gallagher (2008) advocates a consideration of the consequences of adopting one theory over another. Finally, there is a responsibility to communicate research findings in ways which are truly engaging. There is considerable pressure on academics not to spend time and effort on more journalistic forms of writing and to concentrate on the more weighty 'outputs' in academic journals, but it is important to try to develop a civic voice and to find appropriate outlets for this.

There is also some merit in the collective recognition of the many unknowns which surround inter/professional practice. As Donald Rumsfeld, former US Secretary of Defense, is quoted as saying:

> As we know, there are known knowns. There are things we know we know. There are known unknowns. That is to say, there are some things that we know we don't know. But there are also unknown unknowns. The ones we don't know we don't know.
>
> (Rumsfeld, quoted in Žižek 2005: 23)

Žižek (2005), rather than adding to the gleeful contempt with which Rumsfeld's stammering admission was greeted, suggested that he'd missed a fourth term 'the unknown knowns' (ibid.: 23), things we don't know that we know, 'the disavowed beliefs, suppositions and obscene practices we pretend not to know about' (ibid.), and argued that the function of academics or 'intellectuals' was to unearth these. Much of the work needed in this regard involves undoing current ways of thinking and practice, seeking to understand the role of misunderstanding within educational processes and attempting to unravel much of what we think we know (Biesta 2001).

Academics may do well to be more honest about their own lack of knowledge and to position themselves as curious, rather than as experts, seeking 'to complicate rather than explicate' (Taylor 1995: 7). Furthermore, it might be more propitious to avoid a quest for understanding, as what *stands under*, and to look instead for what lies between, or for '*inter*standing' (ibid.: 6),

> When depth gives way to surface, under-standing becomes inter-standing. To comprehend is no longer to grasp what lies beneath but to glimpse what lies between . . . Understanding is no longer possible because nothing stands under . . . Interstanding has become unavoidable because everything stands between.
>
> (Taylor and Saarinen 1994: 2–3)

The pursuit of interstanding involves risking the personal (Ware 2002) because it requires individuals to tolerate the diminishment of the borders which define their identities and their sense of place, and much of the knowledge which is used as warrants for action. These ambivalences, however, could give rise to more positive ways of being in, and engaging with, the world, and Anzaldua (1987) suggests that the model for such existence could be found among those of mixed ethnicity:

> The new *mestiza* . . . copes by developing a tolerance for contradictions, a tolerance for ambiguity. She learns to be an Indian in Mexican culture, to be Mexican from an Anglo point of view. She learns to juggle cultures. She has a plural personality, she operates in a pluralistic mode – nothing is thrust out, the good the bad and the ugly, nothing rejected, nothing abandoned. Not only does she sustain contradictions, she turns the ambivalence into something else.
>
> (Anzaldua 1987: 79)

Such tolerance of contradictions and ambiguity may be something which can be sought and practised in the pursuit of the *something else* of inter/professional practice.

Epiphanies of the everyday

Although the pressures on academics and the quest for certainty which has been a feature of educational practice may have clipped the wings of Socratic insight by insisting that all learning is tied down, there may be scope for opening up learning for colleagues and for stakeholders in policy and practice communities. Specifically, academics could help to create learning spaces which could allow exposure to what James Joyce has called 'epiphanies':

> The epiphany was the sudden 'revelation of the whatness of a thing', the moment in which the 'soul of the commonest object . . . seems to us radiant'. The artist, he felt, was charged with such revelations, and must look for them not among the gods but among men, in casual, unostentatious, even unpleasant moments.
> (Ellman 1982: 83)

James Ellman (1982), the foremost biographer of James Joyce, explained how an epiphany, a sudden bringing into presence that which is otherwise inaccessible, was often achieved through great art, and this view is endorsed by Taylor (1989: 419):

> What I want to capture with this term is just this notion of a work of art as the locus of a manifestation which brings us into the presence of something which is otherwise inaccessible, and which is of the highest moral and spiritual significance; a manifestation, moreover, which also defines and completes something even as it reveals.

Hogan (2005: 91) suggests that this could be achieved by educators, but it would require a different orientation to one's work, which, above all, involves the 'ever alert acknowledgement of the possibilities and limitations which constitute our own way of being human among others'. The gradual shift by public research funders from 'stakeholder engagement' to 'knowledge transfer' and now to 'knowledge exchange' (Ozga 2006) reflects a more sophisticated understanding of the needs of different interest groups among researchers, funders and 'researched', and a recognition of the need for greater reciprocity in research relationships. This shift also creates a space into which academics could position themselves as facilitators of 'everyday ephiphanies'. These would bring to attention 'the quality of what is actually experienced' (Hogan 2005: 92), but which is bypassed because it is part of routine and therefore undertaken unreflexively, and invite a dwelling upon it. To produce these epiphanies, the academic would need to work at convincing the participants not simply to engage in dialogue, but that they '*are* a dialogue' (ibid.: 93). This means abandoning conventional approaches to stakeholder meetings which seek shared meanings and consensus (but which, of course, privilege certain perspectives over others) and creating instead a smooth space for learning (a *deterritorialized space* in Deleuze and

Guattari's [1987] terms) in which partiality – or one's position and interests – is the material for discussion and incompleteness is a specific goal. Approaches such as Open Space Technology (Openspaceworld n.d.), developed by US businessman Harrison Owen, provide a smooth space for the participants to determine their own agenda for discussion. It has been described as 'passion with responsibility' and as 'chaos and creativity' (ibid.: n.p.) and is simultaneously loose, because the agenda is not set, and highly structured, using the responses of the participants to determine activities and outcomes. This technology has been used to try to bring student teachers and students together and to obtain insights from young people in relation to diversity (Allan *et al.* 2009). The approach appears to be successful in altering the relations of the participants and the balance of power and, in our experience, allows 'epiphanies' to emerge.

Retrieving the civic

> I think what you'll find is, whatever it is we do substantively, there will be near-perfect clarity as to what it is. And it will be known, and it will be known to the Congress, and it will be known to you, probably before we decide it, but it will be known.
>
> (Rumsfeld 2003: n.p.)

The pressures faced by the present day academic are significant and the climate of accountability and mistrust gets at the souls of individuals and at their sense of capacity for civic duty (Sennet 1998; Ballard 2003; Nixon 2009): 'Operationally, everything is so clear; emotionally so illegible' (Sennet 1998: 68). For the academic committed to inter/professional practice, the stresses are possibly even greater because of the imperatives for clarity, urgency and solutions, and the difficulties of trying to resist these. I have suggested that academics may have allowed themselves to be defined by 'the disfiguring language of performativity' (Fielding 2001: 8) and may have used this to displace their civic duty. It need not be this way. The possibilities for reorientation by academics, in relation to the ontological, the epistemological and the epiphanic, are significant. They offer a way of recovering the civic duty and putting it into practice in relation to the academics themselves, and to the developing professionals for whom they are responsible.

References

Allan, J. (2005) 'Inclusion as an ethical project', in S. Tremain (ed.) *Foucault and the government of disability*, Ann Arbor: University of Michigan Press.
—— (2008) *Rethinking inclusion: the philosophers of difference in practice*, Dordrecht: Springer.
—— (2009) 'After the break? Interrupting the discourses of inter-professional practice', in J. Forbes and C. Watson (eds) *Service integration in schools: research and policy discourses, practices and future prospects*, Rotterdam: Sense.
Allan, J., I'Anson, J., Mott, J. and Smyth, G. (2009) 'Understanding disability with children's social capital', *Journal of Research in Special Educational Needs* 9: 115–21.

Allan, J. and Slee, R. (2008) *Doing inclusive education research*, Rotterdam: Sense.

Anzaldua, G. (1987) *Borderlands/La Frontera*, San Francisco: Spinsters/Aunt Lute.

Apple, M. (2001) *Educating the 'right' way*, New York: Routledge/Falmer.

Ballard, K. (2003) 'Teaching, trust, identity and community', in J. Allan (ed.) *Inclusion, participation and democracy: what is the purpose?* Dordrecht: Kluwer.

Biesta, G. (2001) 'Preparing for the incalculable', in G. Biesta and D. Egéa-Kuehne (eds) *Derrida & education*, London: Routledge.

Booth, T. (2003) 'Views from the institution: overcoming barriers to inclusive education?', in T. Booth, K. Nes and M Strømstad (eds) *Developing inclusive education*, London: RoutledgeFalmer.

Bourdieu, P. (1998) *Practical reason*, Cambridge: Polity.

Bowie, D. (1976) 'Musicians on life and politics', in D. Watson (ed.) *Chambers musical quotations*, Edinburgh: Chambers.

Brantlinger, E. (2006) 'The big glossies: how textbooks structure (special) education', in E. Brantlinger (ed.) *Who benefits from special education? Remediating (fixing) other people's children*, Mahwah, NJ/London: Lawrence Erlbaum Associates.

Britzman, D. (1986) 'Cultural myths in the making of a teacher', *Harvard Educational Review* 56: 442–55.

Colebrook, C. (2006) *Deleuze: a guide for the perplexed*, London/New York: Continuum.

Corbett, J. and Slee, R. (2000) 'An international conversation on inclusive education', in F. Armstrong, D. Armstrong and L. Barton (eds) *Inclusive education: policy, contexts and comparative education*, London: David Fulton.

Daniels, H. (2005) 'Young people at risk of social exclusion: interagency working and professional learning', paper presented at the Participation, Inclusion and Equity Research Network, Stirling, UK, 20 June 2005.

Deleuze, G. and Guattari, F. (1987) *A thousand plateaus: capitalism and schizophrenia*, London: The Athlone Press.

Diken, B. and Bagge Lausten, C. (2005) *The culture of the exception: sociology facing the camp*, London/New York: Routledge.

Ellman, R. (1982) *James Joyce*, New York: Oxford University Press.

Evans, K. (2004) *Killing thinking: the death of the universities*, London/New York: Continuum.

Fearnside, W. and Holther, W. (1959) *Fallacy: the counterfeit of argument*, Englewood Cliffs: Prentice Hall.

Fielding, M. (ed.) (2001) *Taking education really seriously: four years hard labour*, London: RoutlegeFalmer.

Flvybjerg, B. (2001) *Making social science matter: why social inquiry fails and how it can succeed again*, Cambridge: Cambridge University Press.

Foucault, M. (1984) 'On the genealogy of ethics: an overview of work in progress', in P. Rabinow (ed.) *The Foucault reader*, New York: Pantheon.

—— (1994) 'A preface to transgression', in J. T. Faubion (ed.) *Michael Foucault aesthetics: essential works of Foucault 1954–1984*, Volume 2, London: Penguin.

Furedi, F. (2004) *Where have all the intellectuals gone?* London: Continuum.

Gallagher, D. (2008) 'Hiding in plain sight: the nature and role of theory in learning disability labelling', paper presented at the American Educational Research Association conference, New York, USA, 24–8 March 2008.

General Teaching Council for Scotland (GTCS) (2006a) *Standard for full registration*, Edinburgh: GTC. Online. Available at: http://www.gtcs.org.uk/web/FILES/the-standards/standard-for-full-registration.pdf (accessed 4 December 2010).

General Teaching Council for Scotland (GTCS) (2006b) *Standard for chartered teacher*, Edinburgh: GTC. Online. Available at: http://www.gtcs.org.uk/standards/standard-chartered-teacher.aspx (accessed 3 September 2010).

Goodson, I. (2003) *Professional knowledge, professional lives: studies in education and change*, Maidenhead/Philadelphia: Open University Press.

Greene, M. (1991) 'Retrieving the language of compassion: the education professor in search of community', *Teachers College Record* 92: 541–55.

—— (2008) *From bare facts to intellectual possibility: the leap of imagination, a conversation with Maxine Greene*, Presidential Invited Session, American Educational Research Association conference, New York, USA, 24–9 March 2008.

Gregoriou, Z. (2004) 'Commencing the rhizome: towards a minor philosophy of education', *Educational Philosophy and Theory* 36: 233–51.

Halsey, A. (1992) *The decline of the donnish dominion*, Oxford: Clarendon.

Her Majesty's Inspectorate of Education (HMIE) (2002) *Count us in: achieving inclusion in Scottish schools*, Edinburgh: Stationery Office.

Hernstein Smith, B. (1992) 'Judgement after the fall', in D. Cornell, M. Rossenfield and D. Gray Carlson (eds) *Deconstruction and the possibility of justice*, London, Routledge.

Hirst, P. (1989) 'Implication of government funding policies for research on teaching and teacher education: England and Wales', *Teaching and Teacher Education* 5: 269–81.

Hogan, P. (2005) 'The politics of identity and the epiphanies of learning', in W. Carr (ed.) *The RoutledgeFalmer reader in philosophy of education*, Abingdon/New York: Routledge.

Lyotard, J. (1986) *The postmodern explained to children: correspondence 1982–1985*, Sydney: Power Publications.

MacIntyre, A. (1984) *After virtue: a study in moral theory*, Notre Dame, IN: University of Notre Dame.

Makareth, C. and Turner, T. (2002) *Joined-up working*, London: Health Visitors Association.

McIntyre, E., Kyle, D., Cheng-Ting, C., Kraemer, J and Parr, J. (2008) *Six principles for teaching English language learners in all classrooms*, Thousand Oaks, CA: Corwin Press.

McNary, S. (2005) *What successful teachers do in inclusive classrooms*, London: Sage.

Milne, V. (2005) *Joined-up working in the Scottish Executive*, Edinburgh: Office of Chief Researcher, Scottish Executive Social Research.

Moran, A. and Abbott, L. (2006) *The development of inclusive schools in Northern Ireland: a model of best practice*, Bangor: Department of Education.

Moran, A., Abbott, L. and O'Connor, U. (2009) 'Communicating and connecting: integrated service provision in Northern Ireland', in J. Forbes and C. Watson (eds) *Service integration in schools: research and policy discourses, practices and future prospects*, Rotterdam: Sense.

Nixon, J. (2009) 'The conditions for professional learning', in J. Forbes and C. Watson (eds) *Service integration in schools: research and policy discourses, practices and future prospects*, Rotterdam: Sense.

Openspaceworld (n.d.) *Open space technology*. Online. Available at: http://www.openspace world.org/ (accessed 23 June 2010).

Ozga, J. (2006) 'Travelling and embedded policy: the case of knowledge transfer', *Journal of Education Policy* 21: 1–17.

Paterson, L. (2003) 'The survival of the democratic intellect: academic values in Scotland and England', *Higher Education Quarterly* 57: 67–93.

Rumsfeld, D. (2003) *Department of Defense briefing*. Online. Available at: http://www.slate.com/id/2081042/ (accessed 15 May 2009).

Said, E. (1994) *Representations of the intellectual*, London: Vintage.

Schopenhauer, A. (1896) *The art of controversy*, New York: Cosimo.

Scottish Executive (SE) (2003) *Educating for excellence, choice and opportunity: the Executive's response to the national debate*, Edinburgh: Scottish Executive.

Sennet, R. (1998) *The corrosion of character: the personal consequences of work in the new capitalism*, New York: W. H. Norton.

Sloterdijk, P. (1988) *Critique of cynical reason*, trans. M. Eldred, Minneapolis, MN: University of Minnesota Press.

Strathern, M. (1997) 'Improving ratings: audit in the British university system', *European Review* 5: 305–21.

Taylor, M. (1989) *Sources of the self: the making of the modern identity*, Cambridge: Cambridge University Press.

—— (1995) 'Rhizomic folds of interstanding', *Tekhnema 2: Technics and Finitude*, Spring. Online. Available at: http://tekhnema.free.fr/2Taylor.htm (accessed 19 October 2010).

Taylor, M. and Saarinen, E. (1994) *Imagologies: media philosophy*, London: Routledge.

Thomas, G. (2008) 'Theory and the construction of pathology', paper presented at the American Educational Research Association Conference, New York, USA, 24–8 March 2008.

Thompson, E. P. (1970) *Warwick University Ltd*, Harmondsworth: Penguin.

Universities Council for the Education of Teachers (UCET) (2003) *DfES Green Paper: every child matters, response from UCET*, London: UCET.

Ware, L. (2002) 'A moral conversation on disability: risking the personal in educational contexts', *Hypatia* 17: 143–72.

Westwood, P (2002) *Commonsense methods for children with special educational needs*, London: FalmerRoutledge.

Wilde, O. (1883) *Lecture tour*, Leadville, CO, USA. Online. Available at: http://www.neuroticpoets.com/wilde/ (accessed 13 March 2011).

Žižek, S. (2005) 'The empty wheelbarrow', *Guardian Comment*, 19 February. Online. Available at: http://www.guardian.co.uk/comment/story/0,3604,1417982,00.html (accessed 13 July 2006).

Chapter 12

The pretty story of 'joined-up working'

Questioning interagency partnership

Cate Watson

Introduction

Currently, children's services policy in the UK is mobilized around the notion of *joined-up working*, a 'pretty story' in which policy, generated within the current discourse of 'child protection', is offered as a vision of what might be achieved (and hence what could be avoided) if professionals only set aside their selfish self-interests and worked together for children. The pretty story of joined-up working presents as smooth uncontested consensus, imposing closure, while simultaneously offering a utopian vision based on partnership and collaboration. Indeed, as Filander (2001: 5) notes, 'working in groups and teams is part of the emancipatory narrative of the pretty story', drawing on core ideals such as empowerment, reciprocity and ownership. This all sounds rather cosy, but as Hartley (2007: 205) warns, while such discourses of legitimation appear 'to incorporate democratic procedures' arguably they do no such thing, functioning instead to draw attention away from systems and structures and instead laying the blame for failure to deliver squarely at the door of these professionals. Joined-up working in the current policy discourse therefore functions as a mantra, one effect of which is to cast professionals in deficit terms. The aim of hegemonic discourses is precisely to naturalize and so create a certain taken-for-grantedness. Here the rarely challenged assumption is that collaboration 'will lead to more coherent and effective service delivery' (Petch 2008: 4) and so better outcomes for children. Well-publicized failures of professionals to be joined-up creates the metaphor of the gap through which children fall, a dark well, conjuring all the nightmarish intertextual terrors and the not-so-pretty stories of childhood. Such failures produce a kind of stunned collective incredulity, prompting media-inspired knee-jerk reactions, deflecting attention away from the interesting and complex ways in which 'organizations', as discursive structures, do indeed organize those who work within them, governing the network of relations in which norms, trust and reciprocity, those three stalwarts of social capital theory, develop and operate (see Forbes q.v.).

Concepts of joined-upness, of partnership and integrated working underpin children's services agendas in the UK as elsewhere. In England *Every Child Matters: Change for Children* (DfES 2004) and the subsequent *Children's Plan* (DCSF 2007: 3) 'a ten year plan aimed to make England the best place in the world for children and young people to grow up' (implemented under the previous New Labour administration) placed statutory duties on various departments to work together. The rhetoric of partnership working has continued, albeit within a different policy trajectory, under the Conservative–Liberal coalition government (see Eccles q.v.). Here in Scotland, what Forbes (2011: 2) refers to as the 'inter/integrated policy trajectory' took off with the New Community Schools prospectus (NCS) (SO 1998), a policy initiative inspired by the development of full-service schools in the US which aimed at providing a full range of 'human services' either on school grounds or in 'easily accessible locations' (Dryfoos 1993: 29). The NCS prospectus viewed schools as 'hubs' around which services would cluster delivering integrated services for children. While this version or vision of joined-up working has not in practice been fully realized (HMIE 2004) – with moves now focusing on the integration of services 'in the space that cuts across children's services boundaries' (Forbes 2011: 4), as set out in *Getting it Right for Every Child* (SE 2005) – some initiatives which locate services within schools have been established. This chapter constitutes an analysis of such services, drawing on data from case studies of professionals and agencies working in schools alongside teachers to support children and young people at risk of social and school exclusion.

It has become traditional in writing about joined-up working to tease out a taxonomy of related though distinct terms (see, for example, McCartney 2009: 26). In the case studies on which this chapter is based, 'interagency' working, where professionals from two or more organizations work together in a planned and formal way (Forbes 2011: 4), probably applies. On the partnership continuum the form of working could be placed somewhere between co-operation ('agencies agree to work on a mutually defined problem but maintain separate boundaries and identities' [Petch 2008: 2]) and co-ordination ('agencies work together in a systematic way and may pool resources to tackle mutually agreed problems' [ibid.]).

At the policy level the will to joined-upness presents as 'closed consensus' (Allan 2009: 37) but how does this play out in practice? This chapter aims to expose the pretty story of joined-up working to scrutiny at the micro level. In particular, the chapter examines the construction, performance and interplay of organizational, institutional and professional identities when different organizations occupy a shared workplace in order to examine how these identities are constituted by, and mobilized within, the practice/policy nexus – or hiatus.

Institutions and identities

There is a growing recognition in organizational studies of the importance of constructs surrounding 'identity'. Alvesson, Ashcraft and Thomas (2008: 17) suggest three reasons for this, each of which relates to different interests and is situated within a distinct theoretical framework. The first is 'technical/functionalist' in scope. This orientation connects identity to behaviour and is aimed at improving institutional effectiveness and providing solutions to organizational problems concerning the management of individuals at work. The second has to do with understanding 'human (organizational) experience', and assumes that 'identity holds a vital key to understanding the complex, unfolding and dynamic relationship between self, work and organization' (ibid.: 8). The third is critical or emancipatory, and aims at revealing 'problems associated with cultural and political irrationalities', exploring the 'darker aspects of contemporary organizational life' (ibid.). This chapter is principally concerned with the last of these and aims to juxtapose discursively produced identities in order to examine the irrationality or perhaps, drawing on Paul Virilio's (2007) notion, the *integral accident* that inhabits the spaces between policy, institution and professional practice.

The theoretical frame for identity as understood in this chapter draws on Laclau and Mouffe's (1985) theory of discourse and Althusser's (1971) notion of interpellation. Torfing (1999: 301) defines a discourse as a 'relational totality of signifying sequences that together constitute a more or less coherent framework for what can be said and done'. Power inheres in the articulation or arrangement of the elements of the discursive field, producing meaning, and this provides subject positions for identification. But the articulation of the elements within the discursive field is only ever partial, there is always a surplus of meaning and this renders the field unstable and liable to reorganization. It is this instability that gives rise to the domain of politics as the force that attempts to pin down meaning and so impose hegemony. In Althusser's (1971) terms, identification arises through a process of *interpellation* and it is this act of being interpellated into the discourse that creates the relational 'identification with' that gives rise to subjectivity. Interpellation figures identification as a process in which one is 'hailed' and turns in recognition, the act of turning constituting the 'tropological inauguration of the subject' (Butler 1997: 4). This process is invisible – we think of ourselves as free subjects in a way that appears to us 'obvious'. But this apparent obviousness, Althusser (1971) argues, is an effect of ideology. In the act of turning we (mis)recognize our desire.

It follows then that the extent to which identities are congruent (or not) depends upon the degree of alignment of articulated elements within the discourses which produce meaning; it also follows that identities are subject to rearrangements of the discursive fields within which we practice. Lest this conjures unattractive notions of discourse determinism, it should be borne in mind that in the conceptualization presented here 'identity' – social, professional, institutional, etc. – is fluid, constituting the sum total of more or less permanent identifications within the multiplicity of competing, conflicting, over- and under-lapping, and always unstable, discourses that carve up meaning. Within an organization, what may be termed 'collective identity' (Brown 2006) is therefore a labile and ambiguous construct imbued with conflicts and mutualities, complicities and resistances, resonances and tensions. Identities are coalitions and as such are precarious, always under threat.

It has been argued that the mechanism which mobilizes the relational 'identification with' is narrative (Watson 2006). In effect, we mobilize our subjectivities through our narrative performances. Narratives therefore serve as temporally (and temporarily) constructed positioning devices by means of which we do 'identity work'. Autobiographical narratives take the long view, doing, undoing and redoing self over a lifetime. But the ephemeral narratives of the everyday, the mundane and unexceptional – what Bamberg calls 'small stories' (see, for example, Bamberg 2004;

Watson 2007) – are where identities are performed and re-performed on a daily basis. In this way through our narrative performances we are both positioned by discourses and act to position ourselves. This conceptualization admits agency, but this agency – defined by Torfing (1999) as our ability to act with intention – arises from within the discursive framework in which we are positioned.

Moreover, the positioning that identity work requires us to do demands that we locate our selves in relation to the other, a form of social manoeuvring informed by a range of interests, emotions and moral judgements. Indeed, 'such phenomena often appear to inform the claims of "sameness" or "otherness" in relation to, for instance, male and female roles, colleagues, subordinates, younger and older generations as well as more detailed organizational differentiations' (Ybema *et al.* 2009: 307). Through this construction of the other we establish claims for our own competence.

Methodological approach

The data on which this chapter is based are drawn from a small number of case studies of teachers and professionals from other agencies working alongside each other in schools. Although the studies which inform this chapter included interviews with parents and pupils as well as staff of the organizations, only interview data from staff have been drawn on here since it is the inter/professional relationships I am particularly concerned to examine. Interview data have been used to construct a fictionalized account of the research which constitutes a narrative analysis of identities mobilized within the two organizations. The dialogue draws on what the interviewees actually said (though in some cases this has been altered to provide greater anonymity), but their words have been condensed and reordered so as to highlight particular aspects of the performance of identity, and the 'individuals' presented here are all fictional characters, amalgamations to render the 'script' more manageable in performance terms. This approach does not aim at the transparent representation of data (itself a fiction) but at its representation in such a way as to create 'narrative truths'. Clough (2002: 8), defending such fictionalizations in educational research says, 'as a means of educational report, stories can provide a means by which those truths, which cannot be otherwise told, are uncovered'. Fictionalizations confer anonymity as well as offering researchers 'the opportunity to import fragments of data from various real events in order to speak to the heart of social consciousness' (ibid.). However, while wishing to appropriate Clough's arguments to legitimize the approach adopted in this chapter, in addition, a key aim of the representation here is precisely to construct a *partial* narrative (in both senses of the word). This gives rise to satire, as a means to highlight the ways in which, within the ambiguous embrace of the organization, teachers, other professionals and their respective managers, construct and mobilize their identities (Watson 2011, and forthcoming). In this way it draws on a notion of research in a *baroque* framework (MacLure 2006), characterized as a mode of research that aims to disrupt the metaphysics of closure so prevalent in modernist policy discourses and to antagonize those discourses 'intent on the suppression of dissent, diversity, complexity and unpredictability' (ibid.: 224).

The therapeutic turn

Ecclestone and Hayes (2009) have alluded to the 'therapeutic turn' within current educational discourse. They warn of the 'dangerous' rise of therapeutic education and the 'diminished self' this discourse gives rise to: 'Therapeutic education immerses young people in an introspective, instrumental curriculum of the self, and turns schools into vehicles for the latest political and popular fad to engineer the right sort of citizen' (ibid.: 64).

The therapeutic turn as defined by Ecclestone and Hayes manifests throughout the curriculum. In England this is apparent in the adoption of the *Social and Emotional Aspects of Learning Programme* (DCSF 2005), and is similarly evident in *Curriculum for Excellence* in Scotland (SEED 2004). The embrace of therapeutic education is observable in such activities as 'circle time', peer mediation and restorative approaches to discipline as well as more specialized, individually targeted interventions involving outside agencies and professionals. Whether or not one agrees with the polemic offered by these authors it is clear that a current concern with the emotional well-being of children is a factor underlying transformations in children's services, which can be interpreted as the attempt to develop the social and human capital of children and young people as a means to combat social exclusion. The case studies on which this chapter draws can all be said to be located within this 'therapeutic turn' and so for reasons of economy have been distilled into a single, and entirely fictitious, case involving an organization offering generalized (and unspecified) 'therapeutic support' services located within a primary school.

Following Slavoj Žižek's example, I make the following announcement:

> All characters in the following narrative are fictional, not real – but so are the characters of most of the people I know in real life, so this disclaimer doesn't amount to much.
>
> (Žižek 2006: 33, quoting an anonymous Slovene TV reporter)

A CASE STUDY OF INTER/PROFESSIONAL WORKING

A report of research conducted in a primary school, drawing on interview data obtained from both teaching and agency staff in which it is seen that identity is mobilized and performed around the (mis)recognition of the other . . .

In the interviews, teachers took care not to criticize 'the other' too overtly. Teachers expressed support for the interventions offered, with remarks like: '*it's great to feel that somebody is probably helping them out*', and '*I mean I am passionately in favour of it. And I like these people, every last one of them I have really liked, it's not that I have got a problem with any of them.*' Appearing to be unthreatened by the other, offering recognition of the legitimate area of expertise of the other, signifies the self as a mature, rational professional who buys into the discourse of inter/professional practice, while simultaneously creating a credible platform from which to construct the other as lacking. In this way, while ostensibly being supportive, the services offered were simultaneously trivialized and the outside workers constructed as impermanent, changeable and especially *part time*:

Interviewer: So how helpful have you found the support being offered?

Teacher 1: It's great. Having the support workers here has just become part of the whole structure of the day, well, not the day exactly, because they are not here *every* day.

Teacher 2: Yes, and quite often a child has maybe got an issue on a Monday, and you say right – and they go away and fill in a wee form, and they post it in the box. And you know every day they are saying, 'When am I going to see her?' And you try to explain, well – she is not actually here until the end of the week.

Teacher 3: Janine [the Support Service Manager] comes in on a Monday – or is it a Tuesday?

The other is also infinitely substitutable . . .

Teacher 1: Janine is here now. Before Janine there was – I'm sorry her name has gone – I said Elizabeth. No, it *was* Elizabeth, it *was* Elizabeth. It's Annabel I'm thinking of – who initiated it.

In this way the teachers signalled their own professional commitment and permanence, though not surprisingly Janine constructs herself in rather different terms:

Janine [Support Service Manager]: I see the teachers *every* morning. Like for example, I saw the teachers of two children we are working with today, I saw them this morning, just to check in with how the children were. And then every week I catch up with *all* the teachers who have children doing individual work with us. Then there are other ones that I am just monitoring constantly. I do end up monitoring quite a lot of children, and you do really need to know them all, or at least their names.

Key attributes of professionalism traditionally cluster around knowledge, expertise and responsibility. As with commitment, these dimensions were also mobilized around the metaphor of 'time' as a commodity, with the teacher constructed as having lack of time, a narrative strategy used to point up the greater responsibilities and complexities associated with the teacher role when contrasted with the other who has time to spend and can use this to 'sit with' the child – a pervasive metaphor drawn on widely by teachers.

Teacher 1: And with the best will in the world you tried to listen, and you tried to take time to listen. So it was nice to feel that somebody else was going to be there and that was their total remit for that.

Teacher 2: Somebody is giving them the kind of attention that you would love to give them and you simply can't because either you don't have the skills or the time – usually the latter – and because you have another agenda. You have got to have them on task. You have got to have them working. You can't, in inverted commas, waste time on letting them talk out their problems.

Or as in this comment, constructing the other as having time to spend with the child (and simultaneously devaluing this) while also demeaning their expertise. Here, the support worker is portrayed as a 'vent', rendering the child safe for school (in the sense of being undangerous).

Teacher 3: And he was getting someone to sit with him and spend – I think it was 45 minutes – maybe an hour, no I think it was 45 minutes, to actually let off steam and whatever.

Naturally, the interviewer was keen to establish who was referred for support, but a strange ambiguity surrounded this. The resulting confusion enabled aspects of professional expertise to be performed by both teachers and support workers. Support workers frequently talked about teachers as only interested in one thing – behaviour (by which is meant 'bad' behaviour). In this way, they constructed themselves as interested in the whole child, and succeeded in distancing themselves from the teachers' narrower sphere of concern.

Support Worker 1: I think some teachers might assume that the behaviour is going to suddenly, or gradually, get better.

Support Worker 2: The teacher's interest in, their concern for the child, is particularly the effect that it is having on the rest of the class. It's a lot to do with just not being able to get their needs met in a classroom situation. [**Interviewer**: Yes, yes of course, yes.] Which isn't the teacher's fault – they have got a huge amount of pressure on them.

(There is a certain ambiguity here – whose needs are we talking about?)

Support Worker 1: One of the challenges is working in a therapeutic way within an educational setting because there are two obviously really different aims going on. *And it needn't be a conflict* I mean because in these schools they are very kind of open to us and they are really kind of welcoming about it but nevertheless we have got a completely different goal. It's not about good behaviour you know and then going back to the classroom where it's very much about being good and doing things right and achieving. *So there is a real conflict.*

Janine also constructed herself as concerned with the well-being of the whole child through a narrative strategy that centred on the teachers' lack of understanding of the wider issues (ostensibly presented as a barrier imposed by the teachers' lack of time, but in effect calling into question teachers' capacity to engage with the bigger picture).

Interviewer: What do you think are the main challenges in your work?

Janine: So, yes and also communicating children's emotional needs to staff can sometimes be a challenge because they are coming from quite a different angle. And the biggest barrier to that is not that they are not willing to think about it because they absolutely are, it's the time – because they are really quite big conversations that you need to be having really, and you don't always get big conversations.

Interviewer: No. No you don't.

Janine: And also it's hard for them to focus on one person a lot because they have got all their children and they have got a different remit so – I don't want to make them feel –

Interviewer: I suppose you don't want to make them feel inadequate.

Janine: No, no.

Interviewer: You have got quite a difficult line to tread.

Janine: Uh-huh, yes.

Janine also scored by expressly recognizing classroom control as a key concern for the teacher (arguably the very core of the teacher's being) and simultaneously trashing it.

Janine: And they can share their wonderful strategies with us as well. They help our management of the child's behaviour in the corridor – walking down to the room and back again for example.

While similar themes emerged in the narratives of the school senior management (counsellors as dilettante, questioning the efficacy of the service, etc.) these were performed in a very different way. In effect a managerial self is constructed metonymically as standing for the organization: we know . . . our school ethos . . . our teachers . . . we are a team . . . the staff . . . This construction of self as Organization or Institution forms a key part of the performance of managerial authority.

School Senior Management: There is no doubt that it is very much seen as a key element in school life (we know that from the daily feedback that the management team gets). Our school ethos is that everybody works together as a team. So we are a team. Janine is the third manager we have had. Janine is here every Wednesday (but she is switching to alternate Wednesdays).

Throughout the interviews frustration is presented as a mobilizing narrative of professional identification. Various others attempt to thwart the teacher as professional – in the case of pupils through their misbehaviour; in the case of families through their 'dysfunctional' nature; and in the case of other professionals through withholding information about pupils. (But it is precisely in this threat that identity is realized, the other is the antagonistic force which is held responsible for the blockage of the teacher's full identity but without which identification would not happen.)

Janine: Obviously we have to respect pupil confidentiality, but you can give teachers a general gist. So they might be saying 'Oh, so and so seems so angry this week.' So it's alright then to go back and say 'Well he has been working hard on that anger with us.'

But this was evidently viewed differently by the teachers . . .

Interviewer: . . . and do you get enough feedback about what's going on?
Teacher 2: Well, what would be most valuable would be to have a report saying how it had gone but not vague metaphorical kind of terms about working hard – what does that mean?
Teacher 1: I don't know if am entitled to go and say: What did he say? What was his side of things? Why did he behave like that? What did he say to you? I don't feel I am entitled to ask that. Yet I have shared with her what has happened. I just get the feeling that it's one-sided.

And the support workers obviously viewed this differently . . .

Interviewer: How much contact do you have with the teachers?
Support Worker 2: I purposely go down to the staffroom at break times and I am available and discuss what is happening. It is very much a two-way road I feel . . .

But the support workers too had their frustrations . . .

Support Worker 1: It's difficult to grab the teachers, to have a chat with them, specific teachers, just because they are so busy, but we always go down to the staffroom at break time.

Then again . . .

Teacher 2: And they aren't obviously much in the staffroom because – well they are only in the two days – or maybe just one day in the week and obviously they have got other things to do.

The teachers' frustration surrounding communication was, however, an important part of the construction of professionalism for the support workers for whom maintaining confidentiality is a key aspect of identity.

Interviewer: Are there issues about confidentiality?
Janine: I mean your point about in the staffroom, teachers talk about children. My workers are really shocked by that. And so we have to prepare them that *teacher* confidentiality is different from *our* confidentiality.

Though this was rather robustly contradicted by School Senior Management.

Interviewer: Um . . . what about issues of confidentiality? I mean how are they managed within the staff because I mean . . . the support workers, they draw a definite circle around what is confidential and what is not. And I wondered the extent to which teaching staff can understand that boundary because teachers by and large, although they do respect confidentiality of course, within the staffroom context they will talk quite freely with their colleagues about anything virtually that has happened in their classrooms.
School Senior Management: [tetchily] I don't know. I don't know that that's as true as you perhaps think it is. I would say that people are pretty professional about what is discussed openly in the staffroom.
Interviewer: Yes. I don't think I was trying to suggest that . . .
School Senior Management: [peremptorily, or perhaps questioningly] No?

(In this exchange with the Interviewer we see School Senior Management mobilizing her identity as authority figure.)

Naturally, the Interviewer is interested in finding out from School Senior Management whether the presence of the support workers has had an impact on pupils and the school. Again, ambivalence emerges surrounding the role of the service. School Senior Management is at pains to point out that the best results are achieved with children whose difficulties do not present primarily as 'behaviour problems'. But precisely by suggesting that the service is ineffective in addressing the key (pedagogic) concern of control the service is undermined.

Interviewer: What difference has it made?

School Senior Management: With some individuals – I don't believe with all – but with some it has made a huge difference. Interestingly my experience is at this school that it hasn't made its biggest impact on very badly behaved children. But that's not surprising really – a once a week session, no, that's just not going to solve it. The majority of the individual referrals are boys on the whole, not all of them, but I would say probably more are for behaviour that, yes, creates some sort of disturbance. Sometimes it makes them worse of course.

At the chalk face then, both teachers and support workers experienced frustration in the nature of the collaboration, but this was dismissed and smoothed over by management and constructed rather unproblematically as a synergistic, shared territory, or as one Senior Manager of the support service put it:

Interviewer: You have got a whole load of sort of contradictions in the way you work haven't you?

Support Service Senior Management: I think things might *appear* to be contradictions but actually when you look closely at the strategy for working within the fabric of a school and maintaining an integrity within your own service remit I think what we have come up with is a very well-tuned – at best a *very* well-tuned – model of joint working. Because joint working is not sacrificing one organization's identity or objectives for the benefit of the other, it is a fusion that allows the integrity of each to value the separateness, for mutual advantage.

So in all this we see a complex activity of positioning of self and other at all levels of the organizations involved. But where is the child in all this? For the teachers, the child who might be referred for therapeutic support was the problem child (a construction which invoked notions of time as change, a turbulent flux against which the professional remains steadfast).

Teacher 2: They are getting more and more freedom. Running seriously wild. So many of these children are the ones that come in and they are yawning their heads off in the morning – have had the fizzy juice and a packet of crisps standing in the line – because you know it's all part of quite a lot of family situations we have here now.

Teacher 1: And they all seem to have tellies in their room. Stay up ridiculously late (and all the research is saying that if they haven't slept they are not ready to learn). They are making these demands. P7 [final year of primary school] is a hard stage now.

And the family is to blame . . .

Teacher 3: At the base there is a dysfunctional family, every single one. The more you scrape away.

Whereas the other professionals tended to construct the child as the *client* thereby establishing a distinct area of expertise. The child also emerged as constructed by the range of agencies with which the child might potentially be involved. In this way the child's subjectivity materializes through the discourse of 'needs' in the tiered model of assessment used by the Child and Adolescent Mental Health Service (CAMHS) and as a probability in the discourse of risk . . .

Support Service Senior Management: If a child is referred and through the assessment process we feel this is a *tier-three child* that's an important piece of the work actually and if they are working with a child and the child is the *subject of a multi-agency piece of work* then obviously we will be represented on that group.

In this way the signifiers used to construct the child are set in motion, and through this continuous play in the place where, to draw on a Lacanian notion (Lacan 2001 [1977]), the Real once was, these signifiers mask the fact that what they claim to refer to is not there. The signifiers efface the child while giving the illusory appearance of reality. The child is constructed through practices of 'assessment' by the different professional groups as part of their own constructions of identity. The sharply differentiated knowledges and the discourses from which identifications arise and which serve to construct 'the child' create incommensurable positions. Identity is thus, as Krejsler (2005) describes it, a 'field of struggle' played out over the body of the child ostensibly 'at the centre', but a centre which materializes as the void . . .

Epilogue

Batteau (2000: 78) says, 'organizations more or less succeed in maintaining a façade of order' but 'by imposing boundaries, hierarchic order, and an *ideology of rationality* on differentiation, [they] create a context that is inherently fragmentary and contradictory' (ibid.: 730, emphasis added). In this way, he goes on, organizations themselves are productive of 'confusion, scrambling, chaos and disorder' which is 'masked by smooth talk and polished manners' (ibid.) only in the executive suite and the boardroom. Juxtaposition of different organizations is likely to intensify this fragmentation and contradiction in which 'what might appear as unanimous, routine decisions will often, when submitted to closer inspection, be revealed as the source of all kinds of frustrated desires, unstated criticisms, and endlessly deferred confrontations' (Torfing 1999: 123). The imposition of boundaries, hierarchic order and the ideology of rationality actively undermines the possibilities for integrated working while also shifting the focus away from organizations' disorganization and onto individuals. In effect frustrating the possibilities for the production of good inter/professional 'capital'.

The 'ideology of rationality' is evident at the level of policy formulation too which, as instrument of government control, attempts to construct particular subjectivities through articulating the elements of the discursive field in order to say what, at any given time, constitutes the socially acceptable teacher, social worker, parent, child, etc. Currently, subjectivization in the discourse of 'needs' which produces the therapeutic turn gives rise to diagnosis as a resource to be drawn on – in this discourse having needs becomes a source of human and social capital. As Johnson (2008: 34) says, nowadays 'State power does not situate itself against the individual but instead cultivates an individuality whose sustenance requires constant surveillance, nurturing and development.' This realization of one aspect of the 'control society' (Deleuze 1995) is, however, subverted at the level of subjectivization as the appearance of hegemonic rationality gives way to the ontological incoherence that attends processes of identification. This is the central contradiction, the accident in the gap between policy and practice. Yet this is also, paradoxically, where possibilities for agency and resistance are located.

But the ideology of rationality also pervades much research around inter/professional working. Research in the baroque moment attempts to get away from this, questioning the closures that produce reality. Such an approach might open up new ways of conceptualizing and theorizing inter/professional working that move beyond and disrupt current understandings. We researchers too have our own hegemonic discourses. In confronting these 'our constant task is to struggle against the very rules of reason and practice inscribed in the effects of power of the social sciences' (Lather 2007: 73). But that's another (pretty) story . . .

References

Allan, J. (2009) 'After the break? Interrupting the discourses of interprofessional practice', in J. Forbes and C. Watson (eds) *Service integration in schools*, Rotterdam: Sense.
Althusser, L. (1971) *Lenin and philosophy and other essays*, London: New Left Books.

Alvesson, M., Ashcraft, K. L. and Thomas, R. (2008) 'Identity matters: reflections on the construction of identity scholarship in organization studies', *Organization* 15: 5–28.

Bamberg, M. (2004) 'We are young, responsible and male. Form and function of "slut-bashing" in the identity constructions in 15-year-old males', *Human Development* 47: 331–53.

Batteau, A. W. (2000) 'Negations and ambiguities in the cultures of organization', *American Anthropologist* 102: 726–40.

Brown, A. D. (2006) 'A narrative approach to collective identities', *Journal of Management Studies* 43: 731–53.

Butler, J. (1997) *The psychic life of power. Theories in subjection*, Stanford, CA: Stanford University Press.

Clough, P. (2002) *Narratives and fictions in educational research*, Buckinghamshire: Open University Press.

Deleuze, G. (1995) *Negotiations*, New York: Columbia University Press.

Department for Children Schools and Families (DCSF) (2005) *Social and emotional aspects of learning: improving behaviour, improving learning*, London: Department for Children Schools and Families. Online. Available at: http://nationalstrategies.standards.dcsf.gov.uk/node/87009 (accessed 3 August 2009).

—— (2007) *The children's plan: building brighter futures*, London: The Stationery Office.

Department for Education and Skills (DfES) (2004) *Every child matters: change for children*, London: DfES.

Dryfoos, J. G. (1993) 'Full-service schools: what they are and how to get to be one', *NASSP Bulletin* 77: 29–36.

Ecclestone, K. and Hayes, D. (2009) *The dangerous rise of therapeutic education*, London: Routledge.

Filander, K. (2001) 'The pretty story of development work', paper presented at the Narrative, Identity, Order Conference, Tampere, Finland, 13–15 September.

Forbes, J. (2011) 'Interprofessional capital in children's services transformations', *International Journal of Inclusive Education* 15(5): 573–88.

Hartley, D. (2007) 'The emergence of distributed leadership in education: why now?', *British Journal of Educational Studies* 55: 202–14.

Her Majesty's Inspectorate of Education (HMIE) (2004) *The sum of its parts? The development of integrated community schools in Scotland*, Edinburgh: Scottish Executive.

Johnson, D. A. (2008) 'Managing Mr Monk: control and the politics of madness', *Critical Studies in Media Communication* 25: 28–47.

Krejsler, J. (2005) 'Professions and their identities: how to explore professional development among (semi-)professions', *Scandinavian Journal of Educational Research* 49: 335–57.

Lacan, J. (2001 [1977]) *Ecrits*, London: Tavistock.

Laclau, E. and Mouffe, C. (1985) *Hegemony and socialist strategy*, London: Verso.

Lather, P. (2007) *Getting lost*, New York: SUNY Press.

MacLure, M. (2006) 'A demented form of the familiar: postmodernism and educational research', *Journal of Philosophy of Education* 40: 223–39.

McCartney, E. (2009) 'Joining up working: terms, types and tensions', in J. Forbes and C. Watson (eds) *Service integration in schools*, Rotterdam: Sense.

Petch, A. (2008) *Health and social care. Establishing a joint future*, Edinburgh: Dunedin.

Scottish Executive (SE) (2005) *Getting it right for every child: proposals for action*, Edinburgh: Scottish Executive.

Scottish Executive Education Department (SEED) (2004) *A curriculum for excellence*, Edinburgh: SEED.

Scottish Office (SO) (1998) *New community schools: the prospectus*, Edinburgh: Scottish Office. Online. Available at: http://www.scotland.gov.uk/library/documents-w3/ncsp-00.htm (accessed 15 September 2009).

Torfing, J. (1999) *New theories of discourse: Laclau, Mouffe and Žižek*, Oxford: Blackwell.

Virilio, P. (2007) *The original accident*, Cambridge: Polity Press.

Watson, C. (2006) 'Unreliable narrators? "Inconsistency" (and some inconstancy) in interviews', *Qualitative Research* 6(3): 367–84.

—— (2007) 'Small stories, positioning analysis, and the doing of professional identities in learning to teach', *Narrative Inquiry* 17: 371–89.

—— (2011) 'Staking a small claim for fictional narratives in social and educational research', *Qualitative Research* 11(4).

—— (forthcoming) 'Notes on the uses of satire, sarcasm and irony in social research, with some observations on vices and follies in the academy', *Power and Education*.

Ybema, S., Keenoy, T., Oswick, C., Beverungen, A., Ellis, N. and Sabelis, I. (2009) 'Articulating identities', *Human Relations* 62: 299–322.

Žižek, S. (2006) *How to read Lacan*, London: Granta Books.

Chapter 13

Probing the limits of collaboration

Professional identity and institutional power

Walter Humes

Introduction

This chapter examines the discourse of collaboration, exemplified in the current emphasis on multi-agency working, communities of practice and interdisciplinary research. It argues that while such developments are understandable responses to perceived weaknesses in previous modes of operation and forms of provision, there has been insufficient critical scrutiny of their underlying assumptions. Considerable attention has been directed at issues of structure, communication and professional training, but the potential risks of a 'collective' approach to service provision have been under-examined. These include the blurring of lines of responsibility, the formation of a 'protectionist' model of professional identity and the marginalizing of important ethical concerns. The argument is illustrated with examples from the fields of education, social work and health. In the final part of the chapter, the implications for theories of social capital are explored.

Let me begin by drawing attention to what might be called the discursive field of collaboration; that is, the group of associated terms which, taken together, represent a predominantly positive interpretation of collaborative working. These include the following: partnership; teamwork; integration; networking; negotiation; collegiality; 'joined-up' thinking; crossing boundaries; interprofessionalism; interagency co-operation. This list is not exhaustive but it is indicative of the mutually reinforcing vocabulary which is often invoked when the nature and purpose of collaboration are being discussed. It would be possible to explore the nuances of meaning the various terms suggest but that is not my main focus in this chapter. All I want to highlight at this stage is that the discourse of collaboration constitutes an upbeat, feel-good rhetorical field, increasingly global in its appeal. Writing from an Australian per-spective, Janine O'Flynn refers to the 'cult' of collaboration, suggesting a slavish and uncritical acceptance of the discourse (2009). We might draw comparisons with the language of *Curriculum for Excellence*, the educational reform programme in Scotland, with its mantra of four capacities (successful learners, confident individuals, responsible citizens and effective contributors) (SEED 2004). These capacities have become the unquestioned currency of professional exchanges among Scottish teachers, arguably steering them away from any deeper analysis of the model of curriculum which underpins them (see Priestley and Humes 2010).

However, invoking collaboration is not merely a rhetorical device. It has substantial implications for policy and practice (see Forbes and Watson 2009a). These can be considered under various headings, as follow.

Structure

'Integrated Community Schools' in Scotland represent one example of an attempt to link the services provided by education, health and social work. In some local authorities, this approach is repeated on a larger scale by the setting up of comprehensive Children's Services Departments, rather than separate departments for different aspects of welfare provision.

Legislation

The move towards greater inter/professional collaboration has raised questions about the consistency of legal frameworks for teachers, social workers and health professionals. As will be shown below, this has sometimes led to tensions between staff coming from different professional backgrounds.

Training

Historically, different professional groups have been trained separately, pursuing distinct academic courses and placement experiences. As greater collaboration between professions becomes the norm, so training programmes need to be reviewed. An unresolved question is how far joint elements of training should take place at pre-service or post-qualifying stages (the latter as part of continuing professional development).

Communication

Where the sharing of information among professionals is expected, there are sensitive issues to do with record-keeping, client confidentiality and data protection, again raising questions of legal consistency.

Research

Interdisciplinary research can pose particular problems, with researchers approaching projects from different traditions and methodological assumptions. Multi-authored publications may lead to a series of intellectual compromises – ostensibly in the interests of interagency co-operation – which weaken the findings.

Professional identity

Different professions have evolved their own systems of professional registration and recognition, in some cases with elaborate statements of standards and values set out by national bodies. There is clearly potential for divergence here.

Practice

At an operational level – for example, during multi-agency case conferences dealing with challenging clients – difficult questions arise about the roles, responsibilities and power of the various professionals involved.

Policy

Reconfiguring relationships among professionals has a knock-on effect in relation to the formation of policy communities, especially those which are expected to advise government about the future direction of service provision. For this to be effective, there has to be a good 'fit' between the policy communities and the departmental structures of government.

It can be seen, therefore, that collaborative working is not just a new way of describing what professionals are hoping to achieve. Potentially it could lead to a revolution in the way staff in education, health, social work and other agencies are expected to carry out their responsibilities. This is not unconnected to two other (related) trends, which have already impacted on public services, but a proper examination of these would fall outside the scope of this chapter. First, there is the dominance of a particular approach to management, which has been imported from the private sector. This is characterized by a fondness for strategic plans, operational objectives and performance reviews. And, second, there is the global trend towards workforce remodelling which requires staff to be flexible, accountable, target-driven and corporate-minded. Seddon (2008) provides a sharp critique of both of these trends.

Communities of enquiry and interagency co-operation

Let us now look a little more closely at the nature of collaboration and the various forms it takes. Within schools, teachers are increasingly urged to become part of communities of enquiry with their colleagues, sharing knowledge and skills, and engaging in action research projects. For example, here are two of the aims of the Learners, Learning and Teaching network of the Applied Educational Research Scheme (AERS) in Scotland, designed to enhance research capacity in education and to promote links between university faculties of education, local authorities and schools:

- [To develop] a new model for collaboration among [communities of enquiry] in Higher Education institutions and [to promote] strong links and collaboration with the professional practitioners and with other academic disciplines.
- To develop and evaluate a 'toolkit' for those seeking to establish communities of enquiry in education and a web of instrumentation for those wishing to investigate them.

(AERS: n.d.)

Much depends on how communities of enquiry are set up and how decisions about what to investigate are arrived at. Does the original impetus come from teaching staff, the school leadership, or some external agency? If the second or third of these, the choice of topics to investigate may not reflect the real interests of staff: for the sake of an imagined greater corporate good, individual freedom may be restricted. There is a strong case for respecting diversity and acknowledging that valuable professional development can take many forms. The desire to create one big collaborative 'happy family' is often management-driven and may be motivated by a wish to contain dissent. Thus, collaboration should not be regarded as necessarily benign in its origins or purpose: lying behind its promotion forces of institutional power may be at work. In other words, the discourse of collaboration may mask an agenda of control.

Another manifestation of collaboration can be seen in the promotion of inter-agency co-operation. The argument for this approach has been strongly advanced in recent years, particularly in the wake of tragic events in the UK such as the murder of Brandon Muir, aged 23 months, in Dundee in 2008, and the 'Baby P' case in Haringey in 2007. Despite a series of previous recommendations for more effective communication and co-operation among professionals, these cases keep occurring. While sharing information about vulnerable children is undoubtedly important, it can be argued that what might have prevented some of these terrible tragedies was not a more effective 'case conference' but an individual with the courage to step outside 'approved procedures' and challenge bureaucratic obstruction and out-of-touch managers obsessed with budgets and targets, thereby shaming the various agencies into taking action. However, justified moral outrage is not seen as a desirable 'professional' characteristic: anyone who exhibits it runs the risk of being labelled 'not a team player'. Witness the fate of Margaret Haywood, the nurse who was struck off the register of the Royal College of Nursing because of her involvement in the 'Panorama' exposé of appalling treatment of the elderly in a Brighton hospital.[1]

These initial reservations need to be tested against some of the empirical evidence that is available from research investigations covering inter/professional and interagency thinking and practice in education, health and social work. The next section will review the findings of a range of studies which offer detailed insights into how collaboration is interpreted and enacted in a number of contexts.

Some examples

The first two studies I shall refer to both take a more positive view of current thinking about collaboration than I do, but both raise interesting issues worthy of attention. The first is a study by Nadia Farmakopoulou, carried out in Scotland, looking at collaboration between education and social work, particularly in relation to special educational needs assessment. Her overall conclusion is that 'collaborative activities in this field continue to be limited in extent and poor in quality' (2002: 1051). Her working definition of collaboration includes:

- Crossing occupational boundaries.
- Setting aside the 'rightness' of your discipline.
- Being willing to listen to what colleagues from other disciplines are saying.

She suggests that collaboration can be conceptualized in various ways: in terms of a *social exchange perspective* where professionals perceive mutual benefits or gains from interacting with each other; in terms of *power/resource dependency* where linkages may have been forced rather than chosen but rational self-interest dictates that that is the route that must be followed; and in terms of a *political economy perspective* which looks at the wider legal, political, social and cultural pressures which are brought to bear on professionals in different fields. Institutional power is particularly relevant in relation to the second and third of these perspectives.

Farmakopoulou found that there was a significant gap between the stated advantages of collaboration claimed by her respondents and actual practice. Contact between educational psychologists and social workers was limited and there were frequent disagreements and conflicts between them. But, despite this, claims were made about the personal benefits of collaboration (job satisfaction, support from colleagues) and the altruistic benefits to clients (holistic assessment, better understanding of the family circumstances). In other words, the discourse had been assimilated (the cult of collaboration was evident at a rhetorical level), but there was limited commitment to its operational expression, often for very understandable reasons – such as resource constraints, or pressure of work.

She also highlights the importance of what she calls 'inter-organizational homogeneity', stating that 'the occurrence and frequency of inter-agency collaboration is influenced by the internal bureaucratic procedures of the collaborating parties' (ibid.: 1058). Within local authorities there is generally a strong emphasis on following agreed procedures, completing necessary documentation and securing managerial approval: this might lead to the conclusion that, although there may be differences of detail, the same management mindset may apply across different occupations. However, Farmakopoulou suggests that between educational psychologists and social workers major differences are evident:

- *Different priorities* (for educational psychologists, the priority is children with additional support needs; for social workers, child protection cases).
- *Different modes of working* (educational psychologists focus on the child; social workers focus on the wider needs of the family).
- *Different perceptions of timescales* (educational psychologists were perceived by day-care staff as adopting a 'come, assess and leave' approach; social workers expressed the view that educational psychologists did not take the time to get to know the family and the child's background, which they felt was needed in order to suggest the most appropriate package of services).

Farmakopoulou ends by stressing the importance of acknowledging areas of conflict and providing time and space to resolve them. This requires a high degree of trust – without trust 'there is no sound basis for collaborative working' (ibid.: 1063). She also calls for joint training and for what she calls the 'acquisition of a welfare identity', by which she means that 'professionals would see themselves as members of a network of welfare services' (ibid.: 1065).

My second example deals with the question of boundaries in inter/professional work and comes from Anne Edwards' 2008 Scottish Educational Research Association lecture, subsequently published in *Scottish Educational Review* (Edwards 2009). The particular focus of her article is policies designed to reduce social exclusion. She sees boundaries as places where people can learn but also as uncomfortable places where identities are questioned and priorities argued. These processes are not confined only to professionals and she notes: 'it was not always easy for practitioners to adjust from being the expert who inhabited a culture of specific expertise to learn to recognize the expertise that parents and carers brought to discussion of their children and neigh-bourhoods' (ibid.: 7–8). She also claims that sometimes professionals manage to create learning spaces in spite of, rather than because of, the bureaucratic organizations within which they work. However, she acknowledges that it is difficult for schools to incor-porate practices which are genuinely informed by the procedures and values of social work, because the rituals and routines of schools are well established and often fairly inflexible.

She is attracted to the idea of 'relational agency', which she defines as 'a capacity for working with others to strengthen purposeful responses to complex problems' (ibid.: 10). She sees this as not simply a matter of technical skill but of 'affective, values-driven aspects of professional work' which respect 'the different motives of other professionals' (ibid.). Although I take a less optimistic view of much of what goes on in the name of collaboration than Edwards, I think this subjective, personal aspect of her analysis is important and I will return to it later. She asserts, rightly in my view, that 'work on understanding both general values and more precise motives is a necessary pre-requisite to responsive inter-professional work' (ibid.: 11). How much scope is there for this kind of engagement? It opens up important questions about the relative value of knowledge, experience, procedures, ethical values and personal feelings in decisions about vulnerable children. It also raises difficult issues to do with status and power. As she says: 'Boundary spaces are not benign neutral places. Rather they can be sites of struggle over identity and knowledge and in particular whose knowledge prevails' (ibid.: 13–14).

One of the empirical studies that Edwards cites is an investigation of a policy initiative in England designed to prevent the exclusion of vulnerable youngsters from secondary schools. This involved enhanced pastoral support for the target group. 'The most striking finding in four of the five case study schools was that the academic systems were becoming increasingly distinct from the pastoral systems' (ibid.: 14). This was partly a function of workforce remodelling affecting non-teaching staff and the strong emphasis on academic results expected of teaching staff. Pastoral work was passed to 'welfare managers' who were paid as teaching assistants. It is not hard to see what the effects of this might be on attitudes and status, and the tension that might arise between schools as academic systems and as pastoral support agencies. At one level, this separation had some advantages. Welfare managers were sometimes able to address problems which the schools' academic systems could not cope with, and were developing links with other agencies in touch with the vulnerable young-sters. In addition, some teachers welcomed the emergence of a separate system, freeing up their time to concentrate on the attainment agenda. But it clearly set limits to the amount of genuine 'collaboration' that could be claimed to be taking place. Moreover, although the welfare managers were making contact with social workers it was not clear how social workers rated their knowledge and expertise. In inter/professional work it is hard to avoid perceptions of hierarchies of knowledge – which may derive from a range of factors (qualifications, salary, training, power, professional ideology, etc.). The research concluded that welfare managers were 'potentially vulnerable practitioners' and that 'there is still a great deal to be done to achieve interagency collaboration at an organizational level' (ibid.: 18).

Issues of status are also very evident within the health field, where there is a substantial literature on barriers to collaboration. Research has looked both at situations involving different health professionals (doctors, nurses, therapists, etc.) and at situations where health professionals are required to work with other professional groups (social workers, teachers, voluntary agencies). In one study, the operation of health care teams was subjected to a critical incident analysis and it was found that difficulties arose from three sources: from the team dynamic when members acted towards one another as representatives of their professions; from the intellectual assumptions of team members, operating from different knowledge bases; and from the bureaucratic influences of the surrounding organization (Kvarnström 2008). Communication was seen as the main problem in another study which examined joint provision of services to families where parents had mental health problems, with communication between adult psychiatrists and child care workers, and between general practitioners and child care workers, being particularly problematic (Stanley *et al.* 2003).

Scepticism about collaboration is reflected in many empirical and theoretical studies but it is only fair to point out that some writers are now trying to counter what Hudson calls this 'pessimistic tradition' (Hudson 2002). Martin-Rodriquez *et al.* (2005) seek to identify the determinants of successful collaboration, separating out 'interactional determinants', 'organizational determinants' and 'systemic determinants'. And Axelsson and Axelsson (2009) propose a move from territoriality to altruism as both the condition and possibility for successful inter/professional collaboration.

Clearly the debates will continue. What is evident, however, is that exhortations from governments and policy communities, proposing collaboration as the way forward for a wide range of occupational groups, are encountering quite substantial problems at an operational level. This bears out the point that was made earlier about the far-reaching implications of the discourse. The various elements involved – structure, training, communication, power, bureaucracy – interact in complex ways, that cannot easily be controlled. Well-intentioned interventions may have unintended consequences. Resistance may be based on fear of change or territorial self-interest; but it may also be based on genuine intellectual principle or an honest belief, based on experience, that management-led initiatives may not produce the benefits to the clients that are claimed. The need to be alert to these ambivalences is also apparent in relation to collaborative research.

Research

The discourse of collaboration has featured strongly in research. Capacity building, as pursued by AERS, for example, has promoted collaborative working, partly for very worthy reasons, linking novice researchers with more experienced colleagues. Furthermore, there is strong encouragement from the UK research councils to pursue interdisciplinary research, on the grounds that there are mutual benefits to be gained from working across traditional boundaries. But there is a downside to this too. Think of the growing number of multi-authored articles and books where it is impossible to disentangle the particular insights of individual contributors. The 'knowledge production' is collective and individual responsibility – and creativity – is airbrushed out of the finished product. Too often this leads to blandness, a mediocre amalgam of cautious analyses. It can also encourage a form of 'groupthink', in which intellectual autonomy is surrendered to a powerful reference group.

In an article in *Research Intelligence*, Chris Holligan and I put it rather more strongly when we wrote:

> Collaboration produces collaborators, new cadres of professors and researchers who are disinclined to probe power too provocatively, if at all, or argue for radical alternatives in public domains. Those being 'mentored' into this culture defer easily to the guidance of more experienced academics and, wanting to become members of this community, are prepared to conform, to self-censor . . . the educational research community has been complicit in its own containment.
>
> (Holligan and Humes 2007: 26)

There is another respect in which collaborative research carries dangers. I am thinking of the ethical approval procedures with which we, as academic researchers, have willingly constrained ourselves in recent years – they have provided fertile territory for academic bureaucrats to exercise their 'gatekeeping' fetishes. Once again, the origins of ethical approval were entirely admirable – protecting clients, particularly vulnerable clients, and ensuring that consent is 'informed'. But this quickly developed into a mechanism of control which is sometimes used to deny access for perfectly legitimate enquiries. It is hard enough within one discipline to secure internal and external approval for research. How much harder is it likely to be across several disciplines – especially in areas which are potentially very sensitive such as many of those in the health and social work fields? I can think of ground-breaking research from the past which simply would not be allowed to proceed nowadays, such as John Bowlby's work on maternal deprivation (see, for example, Bowlby 1979) or Frank Coffield's (1973) work on gangs. But no doubt the prospect of bringing into alignment the ethical approval guidelines of education, social work and health is already filling some academic bureaucrat's heart with delight.

Chris Holligan and I said that collaboration produces collaborators. In wartime, the word 'collaborator' was used to describe those who gave comfort to the enemy in exchange for certain benefits or to avoid persecution. It involved sacrificing principle for the sake of personal advantage. Is it too fanciful to suggest that parallels can be drawn with present-day forms of collaboration in the academic community?

Whose social capital?

At the beginning I referred to the discursive field which constitutes the cult of collaboration. There is, of course, another dimension to the discourse – that which applies to the supposed beneficiaries of the discourse, the clients. Its key terms include: participation; voice; empowerment; entitlements; personalization; choice; rights; confidentiality; inclusion; support; and well-being. Once again the list is not exhaustive and each term might be subject to detailed deconstruction. But the main point is that this alternative delineation of the discursive field shifts the focus from the professionals to the supposed beneficiaries. It is a perspective that is often linked to claims about the importance of building social capital among disadvantaged groups (see, for example, Allan, Ozga and Smyth 2009).

It is not without significance, I think, that the literature on collaboration is weighted much more heavily towards the professionals than the clients. There is insufficient questioning of the ethics of professionalism. Professionalism is, in fact, a double-edged concept. At its best it stands for entirely desirable qualities: high standards; public service; concern for the clients; and continuing development. But at its worst, it stands for self-interest, protectionism, exclusivity and an arrogant conviction that professionals always know best. Examples of these less desirable qualities can be found in all the professions – teaching, law, medicine, nursing, social work. I would argue that some of the effects of collaborative working could lead in a direction that strengthened rather than mitigated the negative sides of professionalism.

Take professional identity, for example (see Forbes and Watson 2009b). It is often argued that collaborative working, especially working at the margins, at the boundaries between professions, can encourage reflection and cause people to redefine their identities. That might be the case, but suppose the outcome was rather different – that different professional groups sought to define the core values that they shared more explicitly and produced common mission statements that they all subscribed to. That could lead to a more rigid, more monolithic version of professionalism where the scope for dissent, for challenge, would be reduced even further. If the position of whistleblowers is uncertain at the moment, what hope would there be for those integrated, collaborative professionals of the future to dissent from the approved, negotiated principles of integrated services, particularly if they were enshrined in formal agreements, reinforced in statements of professional standards and promulgated in firmly applied protocols?

What we are seeing in the area of professional collaboration is merely one manifestation of a global trend towards uniformity and conformity of thinking and practice across a wide range of social spheres. We are familiar with the notion of the McDonaldization of society (Ritzer 2008). What is happening to professionalism is merely one example of this trend: set menu; advertising hype; cheap ingredients; and staff who are expected to be endlessly cheerful despite (in some cases) their poor employment conditions. The key drivers are economic and managerial, though the rhetoric makes great play of social justice and community engagement.

So whose social capital is being developed: the clients, the professionals, the senior managers, or the policy makers? Who has the greatest opportunity to expand their knowledge, to become part of networks that might make a difference, to build relationships of reciprocity and trust? Are we not witnessing merely another instance of how power is differentially distributed and how language is used to create the illusion of better times ahead? Will this really make a difference to the family living in poverty, the child whose parents are drug addicts, the teenager with learning difficulties who has been excluded from school, the youngster in local authority care? Will professionals really be willing to cede some of the institutional power that they have built, consolidated and protected over many decades?

Increasingly, I am inclined to feel that the answer to these situations will not be found in the restructuring of services – bureaucrats always go for restructuring as their preferred option – or in agonizing over what 'new professionalism' might look like, or indeed in looking at different types of social capital. We have a society in which the dominant values are individualism, consumerism and materialism; despite all the talk of rebuilding community, for many people a brief moment of celebrity – or celebrity by proxy – means more than stable relationships, local rootedness or ethical principles. All this is summed up chillingly in the later novels of the late, great J. G. Ballard who died in April 2009. I would particularly recommend *Cocaine Nights* (1996) and *Super-Cannes* (2000). These novels, set in the near future, present a world in which shopping malls have become places of worship, in which advertising and television brainwash a population that believes itself to be 'free', and in which the human impulse to violence is allowed controlled expression by corporate interests. It is also a world in which all sense of community has disappeared. In *Super-Cannes* one of the characters says:

> The twentieth century ended with its dreams in ruins. The notion of the community as a voluntary association of enlightened individuals has died for ever. We realize how suffocatingly humane we've become, dedicated to moderation and the middle way. The suburbanization of the soul has overrun our planet like the plague.
>
> (Ballard 2000: 263)

So my conclusion is that we should be rather sceptical of the discourse of collaboration if it is decontextualized from these wider social, political and economic contexts. We should be sceptical of the motives of some researchers who see it as new territory to colonize. We should be sceptical of professionals who seize it as an opportunity to navel-gaze about their own role and status. We need to focus our attention much more effectively on the supposed beneficiaries of all this collaboration – the poor, the sick, the elderly, the marginalized, the excluded and the vulnerable. We need to concentrate on doing better at trying to understand their experience, at listening to what they have to say, and, where they are afraid or inarticulate, helping them to find their voice. Building their social capital is much more important than extending ours.

Note

1   BBC 'Panorama' programme in July 2005.

References

Allan, J., Ozga, J. and Smyth, G. (eds) (2009) *Social capital, professionalism and diversity*, Rotterdam: Sense.

Applied Educational Research Scheme (AERS) (no date). Online. Available at: http://www.aers.org.uk/aers/ (accessed 26 August 2009).

Axelsson, S. and Axelsson, R. (2009) 'From territoriality to altruism in interprofessional collaboration and leadership', *Journal of Interprofessional Care* 23: 320–30.

Ballard, J. G. (1996) *Cocaine nights*, London: Harper Collins.

—— (2000) *Super-Cannes*, London: Flamingo.

Bowlby, J. (1979) *The making and breaking of affectional bonds*, London: Tavistock Publications.

Coffield, F. (1973) *A Glasgow gang observed*, London: Methuen.

Edwards, A. (2009) 'Understanding boundaries in inter-professional work', *Scottish Educational Review* 41: 5–21.

Farmakopoulou, N. (2002) 'What lies underneath? An inter-organizational analysis of collaboration between education and social work', *British Journal of Social Work* 32: 1051–66.

Forbes, J. and Watson, C. (eds) (2009a) *Service integration in schools: research and policy discourses, practices and future prospects*, Rotterdam: Sense.

—— (eds) (2009b) 'Research into professional identities: theorizing social and institutional identities', ESRC Seminar 1 Proceedings, University of Aberdeen, School of Education, Research Paper 18, Aberdeen: University of Aberdeen.

Holligan, C. and Humes, W. (2007) 'Critical reflections on the orthodoxies of UK applied research in education', *Research Intelligence* 101: 24–6.

Hudson, B. (2002) 'Interprofessionality in health and social care: the Achilles' heel of partnership?', *Journal of Interprofessional Care* 16: 7–17.

Kvarnström, S. (2008) 'Difficulties in collaboration: a critical incident study of inter-professional healthcare teamwork', *Journal of Interprofessional Care* 22: 191–203.

Martin-Rodriquez, L. S., Beaulieu, M.-D., D'Amour, D. and Ferrada-Videla, M. (2005) 'The determinants of successful collaboration: a review of theoretical and empirical studies', *Journal of Interprofessional Care* 19: 132–47.

O'Flynn, J. (2009) 'The cult of collaboration in public policy', *Australian Journal of Public Administration* 68: 112–16.

Priestley, M. and Humes, W. (2010) 'The development of Scotland's Curriculum for Excellence: amnesia and déjà vu?', *Oxford Review of Education* 36: 345–61.

Ritzer, G. (2008) *The McDonaldization of society*, 5th edition, Thousand Oaks, CA: Pine Forge Press.

Scottish Executive Education Department (SEED) (2004) *A curriculum for excellence*, Edinburgh: SEED.

Seddon, J. (2008) *Systems thinking in the public sector*, Axminster: Triarchy Press.

Stanley, N., Penhale, B., Riordan, D., Barbour, R. and Holden, S. (2003) 'Working on the interface: identifying professional responses to families with mental health and child-care needs', *Health and Social Care in the Community* 11: 208–18.

Part V

Conclusion

Chapter 14

Inter/professional children's services

Complexities, transformations and futures

Cate Watson and Joan Forbes

Introduction

In this final chapter we return to the complex issues and questions raised in earlier chapters to bring together the ideas and themes debated in the book. We use narrative and discourse theoretical approaches to reappraise the discourses and new knowledge about, on the one hand, inter/professional policy and practice and, on the other, practitioners' knowledge bases, skills and identities discussed earlier.

Previous chapters have explored a range of issues and debates in the context of children's services and the discourses within which these concerns and calls are located, collectively revealing the central paradox within which calls for 'joined-up working' are situated. This paradox arises in the disjunctions in/between policies and practices. The concept of 'joining-up' as a metaphor in/for children's services integration seeks to emphasize its seamless qualities while simultaneously downplaying its necessary concomitant – boundaries, edges, hems – potential weak points, gaps that arise in the attempt to articulate the radically different substances of policies and practices. As a metaphor, joined-up working contains its own 'integral accident' (Virilio 2007) as that which will subvert its own intentions. Indeed, the accident is already present in the hyphen linking inter-professional working, while to omit the hyphen altogether suggests a denial of difference. The forward slash by contrast represents the unrepresentable, the disjunctive moment, the space of the simultaneous undoing and redoing in which 'the forward slash acts as the pivot, the "both/and" of oscillation guards against exclusion, bias or reification' (Manolopoulos 2009: 24). Here, in the title of our book and in the argument and debate presented across its chapters, the forward slash represents the Deleuzian *fold*, 'the complicated enfolding of space and time which entails a rejection of linearity and the embrace of complexity' (Watson 2008: 9).

Surveying the chapters of this book, it is evident that individually and collectively what is conveyed is the complex nature of the task of enabling practitioners across the wide range of services in the children's public sector to work together for the benefit of children, young people and their families. Here we take up the challenge of identifying the key issues that underlie the current search for ways of working better together and so in this final chapter we consider what has been said about governance and policy, practices, and professional knowledges, skills and identities. We discuss these in relation to the complexities involved and the inter/professional transformations entailed and end with a specification for re-imagining children's services futures.

Complexities

Foucault (1984) says that 'everything is dangerous' and, this being the case, there is always something to do – he calls for a 'pessimistic activism' in which 'the ethico-political choice we have to make every day is to determine *which is the main danger*' (ibid.: 383, emphasis added). The notion that everything is dangerous resonates with Rittel and Webber's (1973) concept of 'wicked problems'. Wicked problems are those indeterminate, intractable and complex problems for which a definitive solution does not exist. As Humes (q.v.) notes, the complexities around inter/professional working are not easily controlled and this constitutes a potential threat leading to gaps in services and provision which produce incoherence and hence 'mistakes'. Recognition and acceptance of complexity is therefore requisite in the conceptualization and reconceptualization of services provided to children and families. But complexity can be positive, a moment for openings and for learning in/through doing – if risk is accepted as part of the package of what is involved. Viewed in this way, complexities push us/practitioners towards rupture of older taken-for-granted spatio-temporalities towards deterritorializations (Deleuze and Guattari 2004 [1987]) in the forms of more fluid, less static, reductive and essentializing ways of thinking and doing across the inter/ slash.

Indeed, perhaps one of the most dangerous choices we can make is to reduce complexity to an apparent and spurious simplicity, and to respond to risk in a linear and instrumental way. The very characterization of problems as 'complex' leads ironically to the desire to construct simplistic (though not necessarily simple) solutions that inadequately address the needs of the situation. Everything is dangerous, or we might say that every situation and every solution to that situation carries its own risks – the main danger lies in the way in which the risks are conceptualized and operationalized. Indeed, the current discursive construction of risk that pervades much thinking around 'child protection' opens up possibilities for what might be called the *dark side* of children's services to emerge. The dark side arises in response to the outcry produced as litany in the wake of tragic cases of child death such as that of 'Baby P' (Cooper q.v.). The dark side transforms social welfare into issues of 'child protection' legitimizing systems of surveillance which potentially place all (or at least the 'other') in the relation of predator and/or prey. This rationalization has led, as Smith (q.v.) notes, to an increase in bureaucratic control, placing social workers in the often uncomfortable position of policing families. It is also open to abuse in the covert introduction of unnecessary and unwanted surveillance and monitoring (see Forbes q.v.). In Scotland, for example, policy introduced as a result of *Getting it Right for Every Child* (SE 2005) has led to

> the establishment of a vast database of personal information about our children. This intrusion into privacy – in effect surveillance of the population – is unknown

to most parents, yet is being actively encouraged, indeed sponsored, by successive Holyrood administrations.

(Roy 2010: n.p.)

Roy highlights a form of surveillance in accord with Deleuze's (1995) notion of the 'control society' which operates by electronic flows and instant communication. Through this surveillance, legitimized through the appeal to social inclusion (Watson 2010), 'a new society of *known and governable* individuals' is created (Grek, Ozga and Lawn 2009: 27, emphasis added). However, in an interesting shift from previous policy, one of the first actions of the Conservative–Liberal Democrat coalition government elected in 2010 in the UK was to switch off ContactPoint, the children's database in England launched by the outgoing Labour government in January 2009. ContactPoint provided demographic data on every child in England, together with the name and address of any professional working with them. This act was perhaps more than anything a symbolic gesture, signalling a policy shift away from services for *all* children, part of the government's rhetoric of the 'big society' (the concomitant of which is, of course, the 'small state').

Elliott Eisner (1973) has said that the denial of complexity leads to tyranny, but to understand *and make use of* complexity, new theorizations are needed – deterritorializations in the forms of innovative concepts and analytics appreciative of its elusive nature. Recently, complexity theory has emerged from the purely scientific into the social sphere, providing a potentially useful metaphor for the conceptualization of problems and issues surrounding services for children and families. Complexity theory understands social systems as self-organizing schemata which develop in non-linear and unpredictable ways such that minor turbulences introduced in one part of the system have disproportionate effects in another (Stevens and Cox 2008). The complexity surrounding children's services arises from the intersection of different systems of activity discussed throughout this book, notably (but not limited to): the social organization of families; the complexity that arises in the transdisciplinary and cross-cutting mechanisms for providing support for children and families; and the fluid milieux in which these complexities are realized, currently conceived in terms of global discourses of mobility. It is imperative that practitioners themselves recognize these features and become actively involved in mapping out the forms that future services take. (However, it is also important that these sources of complexity are not conflated – there is a danger that notions such as inter/professional collaboration and 'data integration' come to stand as proxy for 'better outcomes for children', itself one of those essentially ideological constructs that presents as unproblematic and uncontested.) We take this up in the final part of this chapter, but, first, in the next section we examine the lessons from previous chapters about what it might mean to identify with the signifier 'inter/professional' and to work as an inter/professional practitioner.

Inter/professional transformations

As we have already noted, current contexts for inter/professional working are complex and shifting, framed within discourses of modernity which are all liquid, part of the *new mobilities paradigm* which has displaced *sedentarism* which 'treats as normal stability, meaning and place' (Sheller and Urry 2006: 208). Within this discourse policies travel, knowledge flows, data is integrated. In the new mobilities paradigm inter/professional working presupposes an awareness of geography, topography and spatiality. In these shifting and uncertain contexts policy is developed and implemented. Characteristically, as befits a paradigm based on mobility, there are 'motors' and 'drivers' for this but policy is an essentially metonymic device standing for actions that it influences but cannot control and which are subject to numerous perturbations giving rise to unpredictable consequences (despite attempts to 'incorporate implementation realities' [Grek *et al.* 2009: 32]). Policy creates a utopian vision but frequently produces dystopian results.

In relation to changing contexts of children's education, health, welfare and care, three themes are relevant to a (broadly conceived) notion of mobility, namely, *cosmopolitanism*, *spatiality* and *place*. In relation to inter/professional practice, cosmopolitanism allows for the recognition of local identifications and affiliations as these are sustained within broader communities of practice (Nussbaum 1997). The concept of cosmopolitanism therefore offers opportunities for reworking ideas surrounding professional and institutional identities as these impact on inter/professional working. An awareness of spatio-temporal effects similarly offers opportunities for deterritorializations. While de Certeau (1988: 117) defines a place as a distribution of elements in coexistence within a distinct location, 'a space exists when one takes into consideration vectors of direction, velocities and time variables'. A space is therefore an actualization of a place, 'a practiced place'. Transformations of inter/professional working therefore demand a consideration of knowledge/s in relation to the spaces of practice and the identities that these give rise to which take account of changes in discourses surrounding families and, in particular, the places of children and the spaces of young personhood. Viewed as a rupture of 'professional silos' as past forms of doing 'working together', the inter/relation offers a moment for deterritorializations – presenting openings, possibilities for risk and new flows. In the next section these factors are considered in relation to *inter/professional policy and practice* and *knowledge, skills and identities*.

Inter/professional policy and practice: deterritorializations in/with the slash

Not only do policies surrounding children's services travel but the spaces of integration also migrate. As Watson (q.v.) notes, the development of 'full-service schools' in America provided a model for the development of schools as 'hubs' for services in different parts of the UK and elsewhere. However, such moves have not necessarily resulted in the development of *integrated*, as distinct from *co-ordinated*, working (Brown and White 2006). In Scotland, for example, the development of children's services provision in *Integrated Community Schools* was deemed to be 'patchy' (HMIE 2004: v), with problems particularly noted in school leadership and management of integrated services, and this has led to the relocation of integration from schools to the spaces that cut across children's services boundaries (Forbes 2011).

Indeed, schools seem curiously resistant to the fluidity assumed by the new mobilities paradigm, imposing a kind of sedentarism and ignoring the new order. There is, of course, movement in schools but it is not liquid, rather the movement in schools is that which is ordered by the instrument of the *timetable*, 'its three great methods – establish rhythms, impose particular occupations, regulate the cycles of repetition' (Foucault 1991: 147). To adopt a Deleuzian notion, the spaces of learning in schools are striated rather than smooth, bounded rather than continuous. Attempts to encourage the development of 'teacher leadership' and distributed practice as part of post-bureaucratic governance have not, so far anyway, radically altered the culture of schools. Part of the responsibility for re-culturing schools must lie with those charged with leadership, but there is little evidence that this is a central concern for head teachers, remaining peripheral to the demand for 'sustainable' school improvement. As Crow (q.v.), and Cowie and Crawford (q.v.) demonstrate, what is needed is a clearer commitment to 'cross-role capacity building' (Stoll 2009: 124), for which questions of identities across the inter/slash become highly pertinent.

The forward slash as a moment for disorder/reorder gives warrant for new conceptualizations in this re-culturing of school. Smith (q.v.) argues for a shift in the focus of social work from its current concern with policing families to pedagogy in the wider European sense of 'upbringing', thereby demonstrating the utility of travelling metaphors. Can we mobilize this reworking further, repositioning education so as to disentangle the conflation of education with schooling and realigning it with growing up? What spaces can we imagine within which such a repositioning might operate, undoing (heretically, perhaps, even displacing) the school as the dominant institution of education?

What are the implications of this reorganization of workplaces and workspaces for inter/professional learning? Research has demonstrated how 'particular spatiotemporal architectures function as pedagogies that invoke particular work knowledge and behaviours (and subjectivities)' (Fenwick 2006: 289). What architectures can be envisaged which allow the development of pedagogies of inter/professional practice, deterritorializing the silos of professionalism? In response to the reorganization of children's services there is a need to examine the new and emergent places of learning and the mobilities they afford. The movement of services away from schools at the centre necessitates an examination of the effects of sector spatio-integration at governance, agency and systems level for what is done at the levels of institutional practice and practitioner relations. As Eccles (q.v.) notes, close scrutiny of policy and governance *and its effects* are particularly critical in the current moment when governments and policy makers have demonstrated a renewed interest in public/private partnerships, not only in relation to the quality of services provided to users but also in respect of the efficiencies and economies that may be made from service redesign and workforce remodelling that are arguably more far-reaching and radical.

Key here is the need for practitioners themselves across the range of children's sector public services to take the initiative in becoming knowledgeable about what any proposed changes will involve and to remain alert and vigilant to their effects for the *users* of their services. Critical too is the need for knowledgeable practitioners, in the current parlance, to develop the skills of *managing up*, conveying clear messages upstream which serve to inform future examination and debate in policy and governance arenas and thus serve to inform and shape future movements of redesign and transformation of children's services. This concerns issues of professional responsibility, for which the 'passionate attachment' to one's work (Gherardi, Nicolini and Strati 2007) becomes of central importance.

Knowledge, skills and identities: re-imaginings within the mobilities paradigm

The theme of the 'professional' and its related family of terms – professional knowledges, professional practices, professional learning – is central to the discourse of children's services transformations, and, in particular, the flows that connect these professionals working for and with children and their families. The connections assumed by prefixes such as 'inter' and 'trans' mask the junctions and disjunctions among the professional and disciplinary knowledge bases as these play out in transformed spatial geographies across children's sector institutions. Within this fluid matrix the identification of current knowledge production practices for inter/professional and integrated agency working is key, and central to this is an examination of the development of professional and institutional identities as these impact on the knowledge production and exchange practices that underlie the forms that practitioner relations may take in the spaces of integration.

The concept of identity has recently undergone something of a paradigm shift. The well-established corpus of research into identity in philosophy, psychology and sociology (Castells 1997) has been augmented by discourse-theory approaches which view identities as discursively constructed and as historically and culturally produced. In another approach, recent perspectives on identity seek to identify and analyse the interplay of identity capital resources (Côté and Levene 2002) with those of human capital (Schultz 1961) and social capital (Bourdieu 1986; Coleman 1988; Putnam 1995), which offers the possibility of transdisciplinary analyses of the interplay of the socio-psychological, socio-economic and socio-political dimensions of identity (Schuller *et al.* 2004).

Significant in the establishment and intra-professional bonding of professional identities is the 'sedentary' acquisition of specific stocks of human capital in and through specific mono-subject disciplinary knowledge. Such practices do not easily form individuals equipped to bridge and link to other disciplines and professions. Forbes (q.v., 2009) suggests new conceptualizations and analytics are needed to examine the materiality of practices – the forms of practitioner relational networks and flows of knowledge as these are now structured in the new 'cross-silo' spatial geographies of trans-sectoral integration-in-practice. She argues that such an analytic is needed to locate critically the operation of power and knowledge in work relations nd to identify where inter/professional practice relations break down in policy-ractice incoherence and disconnects. A relational theory analytic is wanted to ritically imagine the ways in which 'better outcomes' might be mobilized. Social apital and multiple capitals theory together constitute an analytic capable of locating nd exploring spaces of disjuncture in order to envisage what might be needed in/for elations that can cut across practitioners' home professions and initial academic ubject disciplines.

The establishment of stocks of capital generally has positive connotations (though s Stronach and Clarke [q.v.] warn, 'capital' is a metaphor rooted in a 'rational' model f economics which has proved to be anything but). However, McGonigal and IcAdam (q.v.) argue that *bonding* social capital, which seems central to the estab-shment of professional identities and *intra*-professional working, can act to inhibit ne development of *bridging* and *linking* capital as flows across professional borders. ndeed, as Bore and Wright (2009: 250) note

> A silo mentality . . . actually forms part of the development of academic and professional identity at individual practitioner level . . . which renders roaming across disciplines or between professional areas virtually impossible. Within the silo mentality model, academic boundaries are reinforced by epistemologies and professional boundaries by technical language and practice; the focus is upon the discipline or profession, not the problems with which it has to deal.

art of the blame for this is laid at the door of the discourse of 'standards' that ervades professional training and in which there has been an uncomfortable alliance etween government and higher education institutions in which 'training' largely ikes place. This tension is apparent too in the training of professionals for leadership oles in education as Cowie and Crawford (q.v.) note. In response to this Allan (q.v.) iggests the need for the emergence of 'epiphanic spaces' in the preparation and ontinuing development of professionals. Where should these spaces be located? ideed, how should they be conceptualized within the utopian vision of a fluid matrix f practice? Allan argues that professional education should be viewed as an ethical ndeavour, and urges that educators and practitioners engage in *serious play* in ndertaking this project. Here, perhaps, the notion of 'threshold concepts' and roublesome knowledge' can be harnessed as metaphors to facilitate learning through iis serious play. The role of the academy in providing a space for play is part of its iditional function (see Kavanagh's [2009] exposition of the university as a 'foolish istitution') though this perhaps has been forgotten in the current climate of conomizing and performativity agendas and priorities across higher education istitutions.

Current discourses of 'learnification' ('the transformation of an educational ocabulary into a language of learning' [Biesta 2009: 36]) are pervasive, extending ell beyond the traditional boundaries of initial training, and merging with practice. Iuch has been made of Engeström's metaphor of expansive learning which addresses ie situation in which 'nobody knows exactly what needs to be learned' (Engeström nd Sannino 2010: 3). Located within activity theory, expansive learning is a collaborative effort directed towards an object: 'the learners construct a new objec and concept for their collective activity, and implement this new object and concep in practice' (ibid.: 2). The motivation for learning is held to arise from the inne contradictions resonant within the object. This collective effort directed towards th object leads to 'outcomes' which may then be implemented. Clearly, in the situatio of inter/professional learning there is an inherent ambiguity in deciding wha 'desirable outcomes' might be and even what is the object towards which activity to be directed. These are not ideologically innocent decisions to be arrived at by rational process leading to a shared vision. They are riven by difference – the centra paradox of joined-up working. As Watson (q.v.) demonstrates, co-location c organizations does not guarantee that inter/organizational (expansive) learning wi occur or that inter/professional knowledge and practice will spontaneously develop Indeed, in Watson's sudy, the child considered as 'object' towards which activity wa ostensibly directed (the child at the 'heart' of practice) may be constructed in quit different ways by the two sets of professionals. Deeply ingrained identities constructe around a deficit notion of the other prevent shared recognition of desirable outcome for children, or even a common conception of who 'the child' is, and, as Watso notes, in these circumstances the child is materialized only as a void in/between th spaces of practice. This leads Humes (q.v.) to question whose stock of social capit is being increased when professionals 'learn', that is, work together. Yet Kerr (q.v strikes an optimistic note in setting out a model of practice in which a commo 'object' of learning is identified with demonstrable benefits to service users. Centra to this is the development of a shared language within which different professiona work. Though this has been widely recognized it still seems remarkably hard t achieve in practice.

Guile (2010: 142) refers to the 'space of reason' in which heterogenous episte mologies are constructed, but perhaps we need to re-imagine children's services i the spaces of unreason in which received rationalities as ideological assumptions ai undone in a process of ravelling – a paradoxical term which means both to clarify b separating and to complicate by tangling. Indeed, what is apparent so often is th misrecognition of the object towards which activity is directed. The object is nc *collaboration* or *data integration* or even *the child* but the notion of *better outcom* itself, interventions that make the life experiences of children, in the ideologicall loaded term, 'better'. Cooper (q.v.) reminds us that hard cases make bad law. Tragi though mercifully rare, cases of child torture should not deflect us from understandin that the most complex part of the puzzle is deciding the nature of these 'bett outcomes' and how these are thwarted/enabled in, and by, systems of governanc policies and practices. Here perhaps the metaphor of cosmopolitanism is importai as a concept that cuts across issues around identities. The turn to cosmopolitanis has been identified as a specific capable of remedying the '*side effects* of industri modernity' which has rendered 'basic social institutions . . . ineffective or dysfun tional for both society and individuals' (Beck and Grande 2010: 415). Cosmopolitar ism requires us to rethink our place in the world and our obligations to others. Th is emphasized by Nixon (2009) who urges on us recognition of the 'centrality relationship' as the prerequisite for inter/professional learning. This discourse enabl

is to reclaim the notion of 'responsibility' from its current association with account-
bility and audit.

Children's services futures

The chapters presented here collectively challenge current knowledge production
practices and seek to identify ways in which to recreate them in order to be of benefit
to service users – children, young people and families. The authors speak across
disciplines and professions to exchange theoretical, empirical and analytical insights
and to examine a number of timely and critical questions relating to theorizations
and conceptualizations of inter/professional identities (and possibilities for the
transformation of these) in the spaces of children's services. The economic, political,
cultural and social flows which are currently cutting across and transforming children's
sector institutions have been revealed and critiqued. The junctures and disconnects
across disciplinary and professional knowledge bases have been uncovered and
analysed. Inevitably perhaps, more questions are raised than answered. But this is not
necessarily a bad thing; perhaps what is more important is to change the questions
asked, to reformulate the wicked problems as these confront us.

Key among these questions are what is 'a practice' and how can this be understood
in terms of professionals and the organizations they are part of? What are the
inter/organizational practices and knowledges that will result in 'better outcomes'
for children and their families? (Indeed, how are these 'better outcomes' to be
conceptualized?) Can we hope for intra- and inter/organizational learnings that take
account of these recalcitrant factors rather than silencing them? In short, what futures
can we as practitioners imagine for children's services? It is not to be supposed that
a future state will exist in which 'the problem' will be 'solved'. An agenda for research
around inter/professional working must therefore concern itself not with solutions
but with specifications. These specifications will be contextual, constructed within
the discursive *milieux* of governance and policy but questioning and critical of it,
eschewing the tendency towards what Tombs and Whyte (2003, cited in Sanderson
2004) refer to as 'policy-based evidence'; recognizing the inherently ideological
assumptions underlying 'common-sense' notions of, for example, 'joined-up working'
(a policy largely bereft of a theory' [Hartley 2007: 202]); and 'professional learning'
in which learning is held to be a self-evidently good thing (cf. Contu and Grey 2003).

The issues identified in research into children's services transformations in the UK
countries and globally (Forbes and Watson 2009) focus on the need to adequately
grasp transdisciplinary knowledge production and exchange practices that may
characterize new cross-cutting relationships in *the spaces* of children's sector integration, and in particular to examine the production and performance of identities
that these relationships give rise to. Examinations and debate in this book have served
to endorse the continued need for careful and suitable transdisciplinary research
practices (Forbes 2003) to address the novel, unpredictable and complex issues
applying to children's sector integration. New theorizations and understandings of
the relationships between researchers, policy makers and practitioners that these
hybrid research and knowledge generation practices give rise to, and implications for

all stakeholders of the reworking and reconceptualization of traditional research/practice boundaries, need to be examined. This type of *transdisciplinary* research requires the development of strong external partnerships and participatory networks (Ozga 2007). Strategies through which practitioner-researchers themselves engage in cross-cutting and transdisciplinary knowledge production and practices (Forbes 2008) merit closer examination in order to generate the 'socially robust' knowledge deemed to be valid by wider communities of engagement (Ozga 2007), which require novel configurations of research involving multiple stakeholders. The participatory nature of such research practices and the need for the development of strong partnerships/participatory networks which focus on the integration of research and professional practice in children's sector services leading to a new social distribution of knowledge are therefore necessary. The analyses and debates in the chapters in this book would suggest that to arrive at such possible future specifications requires practitioners/researchers to:

- examine theorizations of inter/professional identity from a range of research perspectives and explore and debate how these might relate to and fruitfull inform constitutions of professional identity;
- explore theorizations of place and space drawing on a range of subject disciplinar perspectives to identify and debate possibilities for transformed professiona spatializations that are transdisciplinary and less compartmentalized and/o fragmented;
- identify and interrogate the methodological traditions and ontological and epistemological positions that populate the field to re-imagine the flows and mixes of knowledge needed for more productive practitioner identities and spatio-temporal relations;
- seek to create research-practitioner-policy-governance communities that will focus on the creation of transdisciplinary knowledge production and exchange practices in ways that are both joined up and cross-cutting;
- identify openings to initiate, encourage and build collaborative research network and openings for inter/transdisciplinary scholarship and empirical research.

Whilst we recognize that the scope of our specifications is ambitious and not without its dangers, we suggest that undertaking the work required to grasp, rupture and re imagine the complexities of the transformation of children's public services is the onl ethico-political choice for engaged inter/professional practitioners.

References

Beck, U. and Grande, E. (2010) 'Varieties of second modernity: the cosmopolitan turn i social and political theory and research', *British Journal of Sociology* 61: 409–43.
Biesta, G. (2009) 'Good education in an age of measurement: on the need to reconnec with the question of purpose in education', *Educational Assessment, Evaluation an Accountability* 21: 33–46.

Bore, A. and Wright, N. (2009) 'The wicked and complex in education: developing a transdisciplinary perspective for policy formulation, implementation and professional practice', *Journal of Education for Teaching* 35: 241–56.

Bourdieu, P. (1986) 'The forms of capital', in J. G. Richardson (ed.) *Handbook of theory and research for the sociology of education*, New York: Greenwood.

Brown, K. and White, K. (2006) *Exploring the evidence base for integrated children's services*, Edinburgh: Scottish Executive Education Department.

Castells, M. (1997) *The information age. Volume 2. The power of identity*, London: Wiley-Blackwell.

Coleman, J. S. (1988) 'Social capital in the creation of human capital', *American Journal of Sociology* 94: 95–120.

Contu, A. and Grey, C. (2003) 'Against learning', *Human Relations* 56: 931–52.

Côté, J. E. and Levene, C. G. (2002) *Identity formation, agency and culture: a social psychological synthesis*, New Jersey: Lawrence Erlbaum.

de Certeau, M. (1988) *The practice of everyday life*, Los Angeles and London: University of California Press.

Deleuze, G. (1995) *Negotiations*, New York: Columbia University Press.

Deleuze, G. and Guattari, F. (2004 [1987]) *A thousand plateaus. Capitalism and schizophrenia*, London: Continuum Publishing.

Eisner, E. W. (1973) 'Do behavioral objectives and accountability have a place in art education?', *Art Education* 26: 2–5.

Engeström, Y. and Sannino, A. (2010) 'Studies of expansive learning: foundations, findings and future challenges', *Educational Research Review* 5: 1–24.

Fenwick, T. (2006) 'Toward enriched conceptions of work learning: participation, expansion, and translation among individuals with/in activity', *Human Resource Development Review* 5: 285–302.

Forbes, J. (2003) 'Grappling with collaboration: would opening up the research "base" help?', *British Journal of Special Education* 30: 150–5.

—— (2008) 'An "integrative moment"? Interprofessional collaboration to children's services integration', *Journal of Educational Enquiry* 8: 20–35.

—— (2009) 'Redesigning children's services: mapping interprofessional social capital', *Journal of Research in Special Educational Needs* 9: 122–32.

—— (2011) 'Interprofessional capital in children's services transformations', *International Journal of Inclusive Education* 15(5): 573–88.

Forbes, J. and Watson, C. (eds) (2009) *Service integration in schools. Research and policy discourses, practices and future prospects*, Rotterdam: Sense.

Foucault, M. (1984) 'On the genealogy of ethics. An overview of work in progress', in P. Rabinow (ed.) *The Foucault reader. An introduction to Foucault's thought*, London: Penguin.

—— (1991 [1977]) *Discipline and punish*, London: Penguin.

Gherardi, S., Nicolini, D. and Strati, A. (2007) 'The passion for knowing', *Organization* 14: 315–29.

Grek, S., Ozga, J. and Lawn, M. (2009) *Integrated children's services in Scotland*, European Commission. Online. Available at: http://www.knowandpol.eu (accessed 20 September 2010).

Guile, D. (2010) 'Developing vocational practice and social capital in the jewellery sector: a new model of practice-based learning', *Learning through Practice* 139–55.

Hartley, D. (2007) 'Organizational epistemology, education and social theory', *British Journal of Sociology of Education* 28: 195–208.

Her Majesty's Inspectorate of Education (HMIE) (2004) *The sum of its parts*, Edinburgh: HMIE. Online. Available at: http://www.hmie.gov.uk/documents/publication/dicss.pc (accessed 14 July 2010).

Kavanagh, D. (2009) 'Institutional heterogeneity and change: the university as fool' *Organization* 16: 575–95.

Manolopoulos, M. (2009) *With gifted thinkers: conversations with Caputo, Hart, Horne Kearney, Keller, Rigby, Taylor, Wallace, Westphal*, Bern, Switzerland: Peter Lang Publishing

Nixon, J. (2009) 'The conditions for inter-professional learning: the centrality of relationship in J. Forbes and C. Watson (eds) *Service integration in schools. Research and poli discourses, practices and future prospects*, Rotterdam: Sense.

Nussbaum, M. C. (1997) 'Kant and stoic cosmopolitanism', *Journal of Political Philosoph* 5: 1–25.

Ozga, J. (2007) 'Smart successful networks: research as social practice', *Education in the Nor* 14: 8–12.

Putnam, R. D. (1995) 'Tuning in, tuning out: the strange disappearance of social capital i America', *Political Science and Politics* 28: 664–83.

Rittel, H. W. J. and Webber, M. M. (1973) 'Dilemmas in a general theory of planning', *Polic Sciences* 4: 155–69.

Roy, K. (2010) 'Big brother Scotland', *Scottish Review*, 10 October. Online. Available a http://www.scottishreview.net/KRoy28.shtml (accessed 11 October 2010).

Sanderson, I. (2004) 'Getting evidence into practice', *Evaluation* 10: 366–79.

Schuller, T., Preston, J., Hammond, C., Brassett-Grundy, A. and Bynner, J. (2004) *Th benefits of learning: the impact of education on health, family life and social capital*, Londor RoutledgeFalmer.

Schultz, T. W. (1961) 'Investment in human capital', *American Economic Review* 51: 1–17.

Scottish Executive (SE) (2005) *Getting it right for every child: proposals for action*, Edinburgh Scottish Executive.

Sheller, M. and Urry, J. (2006) 'The new mobilities paradigm', *Environment and Plannin* 38: 207–26.

Stevens, I. and Cox, P. (2008) 'Complexity theory: developing new understandings of chil protection in field settings and in residential child care', *British Journal of Social Work* 38 1320–36.

Stoll, L. (2009) 'Capacity building for school improvement or creating capacity for learning A changing landscape', *Journal of Educational Change* 10: 115–27.

Virilio, P. (2007) *The original accident*, Cambridge: Polity Press.

Watson, C. (2008) *Reflexive research and the (re)turn to the baroque. (Or how I learned to sto worrying and love the university)*, Rotterdam: Sense.

—— (2010) 'Educational policy in Scotland: inclusion and the control society', *Discours Studies in the Cultural Politics of Education* 31: 93–104.

Index